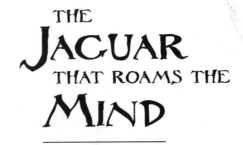

THE JAGUAR THAT ROAMS THE MIND

"Like the twists and turns of ayahuasca, the sacred vine of the Amazon, this wonderful narrative of love and self-discovery connects vast inner worlds of dream and vision, power and magic, with a passionate pilgrimage in time and space. A joy to read."

LUIS EDUARDO LUNA, AUTHOR OF *AYAHUASCA READER: ENCOUNTERS WITH THE AMAZON'S SACRED VINE* AND COAUTHOR OF *INNER PATHS TO OUTER SPACE*

"If you want to know what vegetalismo is *really* like, you could go to the Amazon, or you could read this book."

DALE PENDELL, AUTHOR OF *PHARMAKO/GNOSIS: PLANT TEACHERS AND THE POISON PATH*

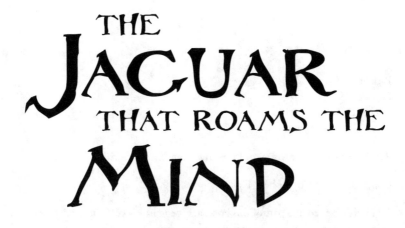

THE
JAGUAR
THAT ROAMS THE
MIND

An Amazonian Plant Spirit Odyssey

ROBERT TINDALL

Park Street Press
Rochester, Vermont

Park Street Press
One Park Street
Rochester, Vermont 05767
www.ParkStreetPress.com

Park Street Press is a division of Inner Traditions International

Library of Congress Cataloging-in-Publication Data
Tindall, Robert.
  The jaguar that roams the mind : an Amazonian plant spirit odyssey / Robert Tindall.
     p. cm.
  Includes bibliographical references and index.
  Summary: "A journey into the deeper workings of indigenous healing in the Amazon"—
Provided by publisher.
  ISBN 978-1-59477-254-2
  1. Santo Daime (Cult)—Brazil. 2. Ayahuasca ceremony—Brazil. 3. Hallucinogenic
drugs and religious experience—Brazil. 4. Human-plant relationships—Brazil. I. Title.
  BL2592.S25T56 2008
  615'.321089808113—dc22

                                                                        2008027396

Printed and bound in the United States by Lake Book Manufacturing

10 9 8 7 6 5 4 3 2 1

Text design by Carol Ruzicka and layout by Priscilla Baker

This book was typeset in Garamond Premier Pro with Rackham and Avenir used as
display typefaces

To send correspondence to the author of this book, mail a first-class letter to the author
c/o Inner Traditions • Bear & Company, One Park Street, Rochester, VT 05767, and we
will forward the communication.

For my beloved pilgrim, Susana

"Los Blancos son más inteligentes," *he said. The whites are more intelligent. That's why they go to the Indians to get healed.*

PEDRO JUAJIBIOY IN WADE DAVIS'S *ONE RIVER*

You could not find the ends of the soul though you traveled every way, so deep is its logos.

HERACLITUS

Contents

FOREWORD

Mark J. Plotkin, Ph.D.

While walking across Harvard Yard one afternoon in the late 1960s, the great ethnobotanist Richard Evans Schultes was hailed by a fellow Harvard professor. "Greetings, Richard," he said. "How was your recent expedition to Colombia?"

"Excellent," replied Schultes. "Very productive. We found a new species of hallucinogen!"

"Just what we need at Harvard—more drugs!" muttered his colleague as they headed back to their respective offices.

Schultes maintained his ever-calm demeanor. He never seemed troubled that his research was sometimes considered peculiar by some of his university colleagues. That these plants often played central roles in the lives of his beloved indigenous colleagues was more than enough proof that he had found something special.

How special is still being determined.

Schultes collected thousands of plants employed for medicinal purposes over the course of decades of research. Most have yet to be examined in detail in the laboratory, meaning that their potential importance to the world at large is not yet known. The magical mushrooms he collected in Oaxaca, Mexico, in the late 1930s, however, yielded compounds that helped give rise to the beta-blocker class of cardiac drugs (as well as the music of the 1960s). But perhaps his greatest discovery (and he disliked the term *discovery*, since he always insisted that "the Indians found these plants first!"), was the botanical identity of ayahuasca, the vine of the soul.

Schultes first encountered this powerful plant in the upper reaches of the Putumayo in the Colombian Amazon. He never failed to puzzle those who sought him out to learn about the effects and potential of the sacred *remedio,* as the Indians call it. Many is the time when I heard him tell some inevitably disappointed psychonautic pilgrim who had gone to great lengths to seek him out: "It really didn't have much effect on me—I just saw a few colors."

Of course, all great shamans have a bit of trickster in them.

I once mentioned Schultes's comments to Pedro Juajibioy, a Kamsá Indian from the Sibundoy Valley of Colombia who had worked closely in the field with the great ethnobotanist for many years. Pedro smiled and shook his head. "My uncle was a great *taita* [shaman], and he is the one who first gave Ricardo the remedio for the first time," he said. "Schultes spent the whole night laughing, singing, and talking in his hammock. Because none of us spoke English, we have no idea what he saw or said!"

Schultes steadfastly refused to write a popular account of his travels through the Amazon, but he did inspire the first noteworthy popular book on ayahuasca, *The Yage Letters,* by William S. Burroughs. Having read several of Schultes's technical publications on the vine, Burroughs decided to visit the northwest Amazon to sample the brew. His account of this experience—in which he refers to Schultes as "Dr. Schindler"—has never gone out of print.

Neither Schultes nor Burroughs could possibly have foreseen how this once-obscure Amazonian vine would become such an object of fascination to much of the rest of the world. Ayahuasca is sold on the Internet;

whole web pages are devoted to its use; ayahuasca workshops are advertised in national magazines; and so many books have been written on the subject that excerpts have been collected into *The Ayahuasca Reader*.

As one would expect, the literature varies greatly in quality. Few of the articles and books are based on extensive experience regarding the use of this vine as a sacrament by the indigenous peoples who discovered it. This is why Robert Tindall's book—*The Jaguar that Roams the Mind*—is such a welcome and valuable addition to the canon.

While the typical hero's journey involves a Westerner in search of knowledge heading to the mysterious East—the film *Lost Horizon* and W. Somerset Maugham's *The Razor's Edge* are two classic examples—Tindall turns this model inside out. He starts in the northern deserts of the Sahara and heads west. The first stop is Rio de Janeiro, where the use of ayahuasca has been incorporated into not one but two state-recognized religions. He then heads west again, participating in religious ceremonies entailing the ritual consumption of the vine by Afro-Brazilians. Finally, he reaches the western Amazon—the original home of the vine of the soul—where he has the opportunity to participate in traditional ceremonies with Indians of the Kaxinawa, Asháninca, Cocama, and Shipibo tribes.

Like all great literary heroes, Tindall meets the archetypes: the Herald, the Shadow, the Shapeshifter, and the Mentor. And he is a wounded protagonist—after an exceedingly difficult childhood, a strained relationship with his parents, and challenges with substance abuse, he is in search of healing and wholeness. That the balm he finds to heal those wounds proves to be a combination of ancient wisdom and beta-carboline alkaloids makes it all the more intriguing.

One of the great strengths of *The Jaguar that Roams the Mind* is Tindall's prose; he has a gift for making his characters come alive. His description of the lovely and haunting Susana is one of the book's strong points. Tindall is skilled at evoking a sense of place, so the reader is right there with him as he moves from Morocco to Brazil and then to the Peruvian Amazon. And he is a student of both history and literature, making deft use of them as he draws parallels and analogies from sources as diverse as Shakespeare, the Bible, *The Lord of the Rings,* the Crusades, and Greek mythology.

Ultimately, the strength of this book—like all classic writing—is that it can be read on many levels: as adventure story, travelogue, personal quest, psychodrama, or even an ayahuasca dream. Tindall has served his time, paid his dues, sought the Tree (or Vine) of Knowledge in some of the most challenging environments on our planet. But he writes with a sense of foreboding: in the penultimate chapter, he tells of oil companies and other commercial interests that have invaded his beloved forest. One sincerely hopes that *The Jaguar that Roams the Mind* will not become the last chronicle of forests and cultures that have disappeared from the Earth.

Mark J. Plotkin, Ph.D., is an ethnobotanist and president of the Amazon Conservation Team, an environmental organization whose express goal is to conserve biodiversity, health, and culture in tropical America by working in partnership with the indigenous peoples there. He studied at Harvard and Yale and earned his Ph.D. from Tufts University. He received the San Diego Zoo Gold Medal for Conservation (1993) and in 2001 *TIME* magazine named him an "Environmental Hero for the Planet." In 2004 he was awarded the Roy Chapman Andrews Distinguished Explorer Award and in 2005 *Smithsonian* magazine hailed him as one of "35 Who Made a Difference." He is the author of several books including *Tales of a Shaman's Apprentice* and *Medicine Quest: In Search of Nature's Healing Secrets.*

1 PRELUDE— IT'S BETTER TO PRAY THAN SLEEP

We should go forth on the shortest walk,
perchance, in the spirit of undying
adventure, never to return—prepared
to send back our embalmed hearts only
as relics to our desolate kingdoms. If you
are ready to leave father and mother,
and brother and sister, and wife and
child and friends, and never see them
again—if you have paid your debts, and
made your will, and settled all your
affairs, and are a free man—then you
are ready for a walk.

HENRY DAVID THOREAU

There comes a moment in long journeys when travel ends and pilgrimage begins.

That catalyzing moment came to me far from the

Amazon jungle and the songs of the shamans, arriving as an eerie and strident call, cutting into the womb of my sleep and wrenching me into consciousness in the early morning darkness.

Awaking in an unknown little room, I cast about between the four looming walls for something to orient myself to. Then my hand touched the young woman sleeping beside me and I remembered where I was: the Moroccan city of Fez. I was hearing the cry of the muezzin for the first time in my life. Taking a deep breath, I listened as my pulse gradually slowed. The call to prayer was not the beautiful sound I had expected. It was more akin to a battle cry than a chant.

Lying back in the darkness, I again felt the poor fit between my images of the Islamic world and the reality we were now facing.

Literary ambition and a nascent love affair had already carried me far beyond the green fields of France. I had come in pursuit of a distant figure named Stephen de Cloyes—a character whose spirit still burns like a glowing ember among the ashen footnotes of medieval histories.

According to the sparse entries in medieval chronicles, in the year 1212, at the height of the Crusades, this French shepherd boy turned prophet led an army of children across France to retake the Holy Land while eschewing the violence and corruption of previous Crusades. Carried on a royal palanquin with the oriflamme fluttering before him, Stephen and his charismatic preaching left a swath of abandoned peasants' huts, tradesmens' shops, merchants' houses, and nobles' castles in his wake. Arriving with his army of children in the port town of Marseille, he prophesied that the Mediterranean Sea would part and they would walk, as Moses and the children of Israel once had, to the Holy Land.

But instead they faced an indifferent sea, and Marseille soon found itself inundated with runaway children. The city fathers, therefore, did not inquire too deeply when a pair of merchants came forward and offered, out of charity, to give the children free passage to Jerusalem.

All accounts of Stephen cease at this point, and nothing more was heard of this children's Crusade until years later when a friar returned from the Holy Land with word of their fate. The ships had deviated from their course and the merchants had taken their cargo to Egypt and sold all the children into slavery.

It was a dark event in a dark time, an age filled with visionary struggles that too often went astray.

Stephen's career haunted me as a parable of lost innocence. I fancied, however, that he might have encountered a better world in Islam than the barbaric Europe of that age. I had therefore set myself the task of re-creating his passage across worlds, and I felt the best way to pick up his long lost trail was to attempt to approximate it. I was joined on this quest by Julia Caban, an American illustrator I had met in Paris, who remained dozing beside me in the darkness as the Fajr, the morning call to prayer, died away.

Julia and I had met at the Cathedral of St. Denis, on the same steps where Stephen had first preached, and we became enamored with each other in a café on the Left Bank, lingering over Fitzgerald's translation of the *Rubaiyat* of Omar Khayyam. I didn't know which was more beautiful, the Victorian illustrations of the text or her delicate hands caressing the pages.

The following morning, against the panorama of the Seine and the arching gray stone of Paris illuminated by the winter sun, we had agonized and then made the decision to go traveling together across the south of France and then make a leap into the unknown by following Stephen into the Islamic world.

Julia was no novice at pilgrimage, I quickly learned. She knew how to smuggle herself into mosques to pray as a Muslim, although she hadn't a trace of belief in the message of the Prophet. With her long black hair framing a Renaissance Madonna's face, no one suspected that subversive undercurrents underlay her beatific expressions.

What we held in common was a love for crossing hidden, and sometimes forbidden, thresholds.

It was only a few months after al Qaeda's 9/11 assault upon the United States when Julia and I reached Marseille. With all the talk of renewed Crusades, it seemed a sketchy moment to show up expecting hospitality.

But then, I thought, Stephen de Cloyes hardly received any, and Julia was already brushing up on her conversational Arabic.

From Marseille, we crossed the Mediterranean Sea and arrived in the Spanish port town of Ceuta. There we cruised up winding cobblestone streets, gazing down on pleasant churches with white cupolas encircled by abandoned medieval fortresses. Then the cobblestones ended. Before us stood a high wire fence and chain link gate flanked by booths of customs agents. Beyond stretched an empty land of pure dirt, littered with cast-off plastics and old, broken down taxis. Our passports stamped, we walked through the metal gate and, bound for Morocco, left the European world behind. We began to run a gauntlet, one that was to end only when we arrived in the Sahara three weeks later, where the desert would prove a fitting biblical setting for my galvanizing vision of a vine winding itself around the Tree of Knowledge of Good and Evil.

I faced the Islamic world much as Stephen must have: disoriented and guarded. I never touched my camera the entire time we wandered through the medieval, walled city of Fez. My hands would pause in midreach, as if overwhelmed by the futility of capturing a true image of Morocco in a little three-by-five-inch snapshot. How could I adequately communicate the claustrophobic, labyrinthine streets of Fez and its sense of *strangeness* that pervaded my senses? There would be the details of, say, one particular narrow ascending street, tightly packed with merchants' wares and avaricious faces, but how to communicate the vast, dark weight surrounding that particular alley? Or capture the massive presence of the mosque in the center of the medina with its many doors opening into one pillared vista after another? Or re-create the muezzin's call by taking a picture of one of the hundreds of minarets rising above the medieval city?

Yet for all its impenetrability, Fez opened its doors to us and we were gradually welcomed into people's homes. The ritual would begin with our showing interest in an object in a shop, be it a lute or one of the exquisite pieces of leatherwork that Fez is known for. Soon mint tea would appear, and once a purchase was made, an invitation to lunch would follow. After that, we were expected for lunch every day.

But there were undercurrents that were soon to surface. One day Julia returned to our hotel looking fretful. She had been visiting the house of Ahmed Lahlou, and she was standing on the roof with his two teenage daughters, Fatima Zhora and Layla, when a group of schoolchildren came winding down the street chanting in Arabic. The daughters smiled at them, saying "Oh, how cute!" Julia asked them what the children were chanting.

They replied, "Oh, they're chanting, 'God will drive the dirty Jews into the ocean!'"

Julia turned white, and then she burst into tears. When they asked her why, she told them flat out, "I'm Jewish."

Suddenly confronted by the indisputable humanity of my traveling companion, the abstraction of the dirty Jew fell away. Fatima and Layla ran off to their mother to disclose this new wonder in their midst. The household adjusted itself, but Fatima Zhora, the serious one, lectured Julia on the Palestinian situation and told her that she could have been stoned for visiting the shrines in Fez!

As if to even the score, a couple of days later, Layla, the mischievous one, thrust a sketch she had done of a young, handsome Arabic man into my hands. My first thought was it looked like a blend of El Ché and Jesus.

"It's bin Laden as a young man," she said, and smiled radiantly.

The eve of our departure from Fez, Fatima and Layla led us out of the warren of the old town into the broad streets of the *ville nouvelle,* the colonial French section of the city. Wearing Adidas sports suits and tennis shoes, the girls looked very *sportif,* and they hissed, "Hashuma!"—Shame!—in chorus whenever Julia and I stole a kiss on the sidewalk.

Earlier that day I had revealed to Ahmed the merchant that I practiced the martial art aikido. Suddenly moving with unexpected fluidity in his traditional robe, he had demonstrated a series of vigorous taekwondo techniques for me. Word got to his daughters, and so it was that we now found ourselves on the way to meet their teacher, Hassan.

Entering the gym, we were greeted by tattered posters of a young bulging Arnold Schwarzenegger and the music of Nirvana. The girls led us down rows of weight lifting equipment and staring young men to the back where a man dressed in a clean martial arts uniform stood. Taller than most Moroccans, he had generous, strong features in the heroic mold and moved with the same fluidity Ahmed had displayed earlier in the day. We spoke no language in common.

Stepping on to the mat, we bowed to each other and began to speak instead in the language of *tsuki* (punch), *shomenuchi* (strike to the head), and *kote gaeshi* (take down with a wrist lock). Flowing through the arcs, ellipses, and circles of the art, as we shared techniques we also learned trust and the qualities of each other's minds. Becoming bolder and improvisatory, we began laughing at miscues and taking high falls. After an hour, Julia stepped in and reminded me we had a bus to catch. Hassan and I bid each other farewell, embracing as brothers, brought together by an art founded in Japan after World War II to bring harmony as a martial principle into the conflicts of the world.

Leaving the medieval city and heading south we crossed the snowy Atlas Mountains, our bus arriving sheathed in ice at the summit. There we left the Mediterranean world behind, descending into a landscape of the purest stone and dust, broken only by the emerald green of palms when the road followed the contour of a river.

Journeying day after day into the Draa Valley, we watched complexions turn from light brown to black and figures disappear beneath swathing. Across a landscape that had suddenly opened like a shutter, the interior of Africa loomed.

I wondered how such an absolutely flat landscape would have appeared to a young French shepherd from a terrain of rolling green hills and limestone outcroppings. Would he have thought he had come to the end of the world?

Arriving in the Moroccan city of Tamegroute, we found that a deep blue, parched sky attended each day and the nights were desert clear. Even the labyrinthine, walled settlements were constructed of earth, blending into the endless expanses as if all were either earth or sky. Nothing intruded on this isolation—no trees, no clouds, no birds, or human decoration of any kind. The women passed by in veiled silhouettes, and the men sat draped in their pointy-hooded *jelabas* in the coolness of the shade. Children would present the family dog to us as Bush (dogs are given particularly low esteem in Islamic countries), and then mimic the sound of bombs falling from the sky. While I wrote in my journal, others nearby passed the still hours chanting the Koran.

Julia and I had come to Tamegroute to visit a Sufi library of medieval manuscripts. What we got was a brief glimpse at exquisite calligraphic and scientific works, observed through panes of glass while the sharif shouted in our ears "astronomical work!" or "descendants of Mohammed!" and tried to hustle us along so he could go to prayer.

To find that one could survive amidst such extraordinary textures of sound and color, even under the habitual glare of Islamic culture, was exhilarating. In the darkness of the mornings I arose to the Fajr, the muezzin's cry of "God is great," agreeing with him that "It is better to pray than sleep."

The honeymoon abruptly ended one day. Roaming as Stephen through the chilly, narrow maze of Tamegroute's earthen streets, I emerged into an open space with a dusty water fountain (also fashioned of mud). Encountering a small group of old men sitting in the road, I wished them good day. They returned my greeting. Walking on I found, close by, an opening in the wall, and looking in I saw a green wooden doorway carved with geometric designs, with an internal door in the shape of a mihrab.*

Surprised to see it ensconced like a hobbit door in the earthen wall, I walked toward it, and entering, I encountered a small mosque. Prayer

---

*Typically a mihrab is a niche set into the middle of the wall of a building in order to indicate the direction of Mecca.

mats lined the floor between the pillars and a couple pairs of *babouches* (pointy-toed slippers) sat facing toward the center of the room. The place was strikingly austere, somber, dark. Drawn toward an adjacent doorway, I saw a well for ritual purification.

A single beam of light illuminated the interior. The eternal stillness of the desert was in the room. It was the same well that Abraham, Isaac, and Jacob had drawn from, unchanged by the least movement of time.

Standing transfixed on the threshold, I became aware that the old men were filing into prayer behind me. I turned. As they laid eyes upon me—the blue-eyed infidel near the sacred space—their faces blanched. There was much angry gesticulation and baleful staring, and I realized that I had caused offense not simply because I had not performed the required ablutions or because I was non-Muslim, but because I was essentially unclean, like a pig, and needed to be driven away.

My aikido training abandoned me. Instead of declaring "Allah akbar" and bowing on the spot toward Mecca, I extricated myself with apologies.

It was a bad move. Going out into the street, I was quickly picked out by a small group of hostile schoolchildren and found myself surrounded by them. A little girl hefted a heavy skull-cracker of a stone and threatened to cast it at me, her face deeply ugly with the violence of our primate species. Looking into her eyes, I saw no reflection back. Through my adrenaline haze, I dimly realized that this experience also was as old as Abraham, Isaac, and Jacob.

Leveling my finger at the girl's face, I said, *"No!"* and held her gaze with mine. The stone was lowered. Stepping into a doorway, I waited for the children to disperse, and then I walked shakily back to my hotel room. There, sitting on the edge of my bed, I felt the ancient hatreds of our species. From the rulers of nations casting smart bombs to children hefting stones in dust-choked villages, the dark inheritance of intertribal aggression lay exposed like an archaeological stratum in this land.

I had stumbled upon the fundament. "This is as far into timeless biblical culture as I wish to go for the moment, thank you," I concluded out loud. It was time to take evasive action.

Julia and I headed east, toward the Sahara and the home of the more tolerant desert tribes. Arriving in Errachidia, we encountered a strip of hotels where the great waves of sand, the *ergs,* of the Saharan desert lap up on the border with Algeria. But we had run the gauntlet in Fez only to get conned again.

After an initial foray into the dunes, I came back intoxicated and agreed to hire three camels and a guide to lead us on a five-day jaunt into the desert. The owner of our hotel, Ibrahim, attempted to get us stoned on hashish and kept repeating the word *tranque* (an amalgam of "no problem" and "mellow out") as a mantra while hypnotizing me into paying him large amounts of money for this desert fantasy.

The next morning we faced reality. The camels were authentic, no doubt, but we weren't precisely going to *ride* them. We were going to be *led* on them by a boy named Ahmed who was missing a front tooth and wore brilliant yellow boots. In other words, he was going to walk us on a leash. Even *he* didn't know how to control a camel from camelback. Julia whirled on me with accusatory eyes. Our relationship had also left the honeymoon stage, and we had just spent a tense night.

"I'm sorry," I said, my images of roaming like a wild Bedouin biting the dust. "I didn't know." I promised to pay for the adventure.

We mounted, but as we passed through the village we felt ashamed of looking like the tourists we had revealed ourselves to be and got back off.

Out in the desert, Ahmed dubbed us Mohammad and Fatima, and he turned out to be completely at home. We came to admire him. I learned how to make a snorting and roaring camel settle down to a folded position in the sand with repeated commands of "Ooch! Ooch!" and I struggled in vain to ward off the rogue camels who came raiding our camels' food. We met young shepherd boys with their flocks of goats, and soldiers guarding the emptiness that borders Morocco from the emptiness that borders Algeria, who proudly showed us around their oasis. We sat wrapped in blankets by the fire at night and ate *tagine* while taking in the desert stars.

I took to riding my camel occasionally. Julia refused to ride after nearly being thrown by hers. One morning as she walked alongside me she looked up at me swaying upon my mount and commented acidly, "Lawrence of Inania."

Visions, dreams, and prophetic inspirations still come in the desert. As we moved to the sound of our camels' padded feet breaking the crust of the earth, through the calm stretches and turbulent swells of the greatest mineral sea on the planet, we began to lose our habitual assumption of our place in the cosmos.

Paul Bowles, an expatriate American who wrote much on the North African desert, once told a story about the fresh recruits to the Foreign Legion. Arriving boys with open and naive faces, one day, a mere sand dune away from the camp, they experienced the setting of the sun and the rising of the stars. They then knew they were entirely alone in the universe. The veterans, seeing the set of their faces changed when they returned to camp, nodded among themselves and commented, "Ah, the Baptism of Solitude."

And so one day, as I rode my camel a vision came to me.

Unlike Saul on the road to Damascus, I wasn't knocked off my mount and blinded. Nonetheless, I was keenly aware the Muse wished me to take up and write. I, in my role as financial backer of the expedition, called a halt and went and sat on my own beneath a palm tree. By then, other characters from Stephen's story had appeared to me, one of them modeled after the English explorer and mystic Sir Richard Burton. Sitting in my patch of shade, I transcribed these words of instruction that he had passed on to the young Stephen:

For every poisonous and harmful thing that grows upon the earth, God has placed a medicine as an antidote. And as we know, there is often a symbiotic relation between the two. Close to the hurt lies growing the balm. As it is upon earth, so it was in paradise. Winding among the boughs of the Tree of Knowledge was a vine, a creature wise like the serpent and gifted with the antidote to the poison of knowledge of good and evil within the apple. Before Adam and his family were driven forth, Gabriel had pity upon them, and gave them a shoot of the vine, telling them that while Eden was now barred to them, the effects of the apple's toxins could be counteracted by a preparation made from the vine. Drinking would produce the experience of bodily death, without the mortal effects. Instead, it would be the self with its delusions of greed, hatred, and ignorance, brought into being by the bite of the apple, which would die. It was a dire remedy to open the mind to the wisdom of the creator once again. Adam took it without fully comprehending its significance, being but newly come into mankind's terrible inheritance, and he planted it in Canaan.

Yes, I thought. If only we could find the antidote to whatever it was our ancestors once ate: this toxin that blinds us to our deep communion with one another—across species, across genera, across hierarchies of divine and earthly. Who are we to arrogate the power to declare ourselves isolated from the rest of the universe? Who are we to set up this San Quentin Prison of the human mind?

I had heard luminous tales of such a vine growing in the deep jungle, where stars silhouette the trees above, water is alive, and the earth pulses with a light that seems to glow of its own. I had heard also of the shamans who sing to the vine and direct its healing powers. If such medicines existed to counteract the poison, could we not enter into an original dreamtime, a radical condition that existed before the eating of the fatal fruit? Would not such a perspective heal us at the root of our sickness, instead of merely doctoring the branches?

In the middle of the planet's greatest desert, a new road beckoned, this one leading to the wet fecundity of the greatest rain forest on earth.

Leaving Errachidia, Julia and I traveled to Marrakesh, where the mounting tensions between us drove us our separate ways, the ideal images of the *Rubaiyat* that we had treasured within us broken. She stayed on to apprentice with a painter of traditional designs while I caught an overnight train to Casablanca and boarded an early-morning ship across the Straits of Gibraltar.

Standing on the windy deck midway between Africa and Europe in the sunshine of a new day, I felt my pilgrimage had failed. I had not crossed the threshold into another culture, nor had I resurrected Stephen de Cloyes. Staring into the primitive face of our hatreds had been an epiphany, an enigmatic revelation not just of the world's disease, but of my own as well. Yet a seed had been planted in me by the vision in the Sahara, whose growth would spur my subsequent journey to the rain forest and be recounted in the pages of this book.

Awaking the next morning in the Spanish port town of Algeciras to the sound of church bells, I walked toward the church whose founder had taught "Love your enemy," now keenly aware that the soil I crossed was steeped with the blood of Christians and Muslims alike. I realized that the sweetly ringing bells were every bit as much of a war cry as the call of the muezzin. Attending a morning Mass before an enthroned Christ, I reflected that all our modernity, secularism, humanism, science, and technology are mere ornaments overlaid upon that figure carved in wood upon the altar.

Leaving the church, I crossed the street and walked right into the path of an oncoming motorcycle.

The vehicle swerved and managed only to sideswipe me, but the helmet of the second passenger delivered a smart rap to my face and I saw black for a few moments. When my sight cleared it was to the image of the motorcycle disappearing down the road, its rear passenger angrily shaking his fist at me.

Stumbling over to the opposite sidewalk, I sat on the curb nursing my bleeding nose. This was the final blow. I'd had enough of following around the vanished tracks of some kid visionary from the Middle Ages. It was time to follow my own vision and make my pilgrimage to the Amazon jungle.

2 THE JAGUAR that ROAMS the MIND

The depths of mind, the unconscious, are our inner wilderness areas, and that is where a bobcat is right now. I do not mean personal bobcats in personal psyches, but the bobcat that roams from dream to dream.

GARY SNYDER

The people of Rio de Janeiro call themselves Cariocas. They are the only people I know of who call themselves a name given to them by those they conquered, those who looked into their world from the outside and named it. Carioca. White Man's House.

Newly arrived in Brazil, I sit in a sidewalk café watching an immaculately dressed, older black man with silvered hair and a gold ring on his finger. Swept up in a great passion, he gestures expansively with his tiny hands, gathering in and then driving away his audience, his face waxing ecstatic and waning melancholic, like a singer of tango spinning out his bittersweet themes.

Problem is, there is no one seated at his table. He is talking to thin air.

Even from here you can feel the heart of the world, the Amazon, I think. Yet here we are, cast up on these shores from our own wrecked dream, where like televisions left on in an empty room, we talk. I look up at the canopy of the café and suspect that it and the gritty roar of traffic and the aggressive buzz of conversation could fade in an instant, and I would awaken beneath a forest canopy, the sunlight penetrating through, in pure silence, to find I had been dreaming like the old man, but my dream had been Western civilization.

Upon returning to California from Morocco, I settled back into the old hunter's cabin I occupied in the foothills of the Sierra Nevada, located down winding dirt roads on a ridge above the Yuba River. Between driving my old pickup truck down to teach in the valley and working the land, I commenced my research into the healing vine I had seen in the Saharan desert.

The vine, I learned, grows throughout the vast Amazonian rain basin. In Quechua, the language of the original Incas, it is called *ayahuasca,* a word that seems to coil itself around the tongue when spoken. Its etymology couldn't be clearer: *aya* means "spirit," "ancestor," or "dead person," and *huasca,* "vine" or "rope." Ayahuasca is the vine of the spirits.

Ethnobotanists estimate the medicinal and shamanic use of the vine among the Amazonian tribes goes back for millennia. How far back no one really knows for sure. What is certain, however, is that it began its emergence from the forest into the modern state of Brazil in the 1930s in the hands of Irineu Serra. Irineu was a Brazilian soldier and rubber tapper who, participating in tribal ceremonies in Peru, had a vision of a woman in the moon who identified herself as the queen of the forest, a being he later understood as an emanation of the divine feminine. She sent him into the forest to fast and pray and drink the "tea," and he came forth an *iluminado,* "like Jesus, like Buddha," I was later told at one of the churches Mestre (Master) Irineu founded.

This curious tea came to be known as *daime* in Brazil, meaning "give me," after the initial word of many of the prayers in the Christian communities founded by the Mestre: give me faith, give me love, give me strength. . . .

I also learned that the medicine is actually a mixture of two plants, whose chemical synergy is so precise, and the effects evoked so specialized, that the odds of its having been discovered through trial and error seem astronomically unlikely to ethnobotanists. The ayahuasca vine (*Banisteriopsis caapi*) contains alkaloids called harmine, harmaline, and tetrahydroharmine—those exotic, often poisonous, often medicinal, molecules produced at the higher end of plant evolution. These indole alkaloids form a remarkable partnership with the ingredients of another plant called chacruna (*Psychotria viridia*), which contains the vision-inducing alkaloid DMT, or dimethyltryptamine, a widely and naturally occurring alkaloid also present in bananas and pineapples.

DMT is also naturally produced by the human organism, and it is so similar to serotonin in its makeup that it utilizes the receptors of the brain normally reserved for serotonin. And DMT would flood in, except for one fact. The body also produces monoamine oxidase (MAO), which occurs in high concentrations in the blood, stomach, and liver to break down the vision-inducing DMT.

This is one of the places where the remarkable synergy of the two plants comes into play, I learned. The harmaline contained by ayahuasca actually inhibits the MAOs from breaking down DMT, allowing high levels of DMT to reach the serotonin receptors of the brain.

One thing is certain. The brain is hungry for DMT, and it actively transports it across the highly selective blood-brain barrier when it can find it. One major research study of DMT suggests, with a high degree of speculation, that it is the pineal gland—Rene Descartes's seat of the soul—that produces DMT, and that this gland floods the organism with DMT at times of biological transition: birth, death, giving birth, or severe illness.*

---

*See Rick Strassman's *DMT: The Spirit Molecule* for more about the role of this intriguing alkaloid.

This possibility offers biological insights into accounts of mystical experiences, such as Julian of Norwich's "Showings" of the divinity of Christ,* experiences remarkably reminiscent of the opening of the gates of the soul that come from drinking this strange brew.†

In my quest for a setting in which to experience ayahuasca, all paths had converged on Philippe Bandeira de Melo, a Jungian psychologist who welcomed me to his "inter-religious center," the Arca da Criacão, to take the sacrament of his community.

So it was, half a year after my return from the Mediterrean, I found myself in a suburb of Rio wondering what I had now gotten myself into. My first impression as I wandered through the Arca was it looked like the front of a Mexican bus. Within the "Ark of Creation," figures of austere Byzantine saints rubbed shoulders with lavish, multiarmed Hindu deities. Buddhas sat with Taoist symbols in their laps. Sri Aurobindo, Sai Baba, and other saints of India gazed from the walls. The altar, abided over by Christ, his hand upraised in benediction, was festooned with Islamic calligraphy, winged Egyptian gods, shamans' drums, Aztec princes of flowers, animal totems, Taoist Immortals, Native Americans wearing feather headdresses, and, finally, the psychologist Carl Jung.

It looked like the whole procession of humankind's religious expression had filed in there and hunkered down to accompany the spiritual voyages of this community. Walking out onto the courtyard, I found a huge tile cross that could be lit up like a Christmas tree in the night. Below lay the fabled city of Rio, with its familiar landmarks, beaches, and high rises, lazily circled by jumbo jets. As I nervously awaited my first meeting with Philippe, I realized the Arca felt like a spiritual playroom for adults, with sacred toys strewn about everywhere. It gave me a good feeling.

Philippe appeared in slippers, wearing khakis and a T-shirt, gazing

---

*Julian of Norwich (ca. 1342–1416) was an English mystic who had a series of extraordinary visions that she recorded in her work, *Sixteen Revelations of Divine Love.*

†I also discovered that DMT is listed on the government's Schedule I of the Controlled Substances Act (CSA). In other words, it ranks up there with LSD as a dangerous substance, in the watchful eyes of the U.S. government.

at me over half-moon reading glasses balanced on the tip of his nose. Big and loose-limbed like a bear, of European descent, he shook my hand and invited me, in Spanish, to sit and have tea with him. He had the sniffles, and he interspersed our conversation with a sound like a straw probing the bottom of a near-emptied glass.

"Did you make it here okay?" he inquired.

"Actually, the driver tried to lie to me about what neighborhood we were in and we almost got in a fight."

"Be very careful in Rio. People here smile a lot, love to dance and sing, but beneath the surface is desperation. You can hear automatic weapon fire from the *favela*—the shantytown—across the valley almost every night."

It was true. Only the night before I had heard the terrible sound of a gun, fired repeatedly, probingly, almost meditatively. Then after some minutes I heard the beeps of a police car investigating the scene, its electronic murmuring audible in the sudden silence that had fallen. I had felt for the first time that visceral fear of stray bullets shared by all Cariocas.

Leaving behind the theme of survival in Rio, we turned to the work of the Arca.

Knowing I was out of my depth, I asked if the Arca was working to blend the different religious traditions of the planet.

"What we are doing here is not syncretism, but an organic synthesis," Philippe explained. "We sing the songs of the Evangelicals, the Catholics, and the Afro-indigenous religions in our ceremonies. No religious expression is excluded."

Songs were key, that was clear. I decided to wait to experience the work before inquiring further. The next *trabalho,* or work, of the community would be Christmas day, and I was welcome to attend. Philippe, I learned that morning, was a devout storyteller. And as a follower of Carl Jung, he had great faith in the curative powers within darkness: the womb, the tomb, the place where the seed sprouts, the dream. Even madness.

He began his work as a disciple of Nise da Silveira, who, dissatisfied with the methodologies being used for the treatment of the insane (the majority of patients in Rio lay comatose between electroshock sessions or drug treatments), began what can only be described as a form of spiritual community, the Casa das Palmeiras, within the sprawling mental hospital of Rio de Janeiro. There were no bars, the doors were never locked, and patients were given complete freedom of expression inside the Casa. Nor was there a distinction between doctors and patients. Like medieval monks, all wore a common garb, and all engaged in a single activity: art.

The therapeutic principle underlying the institution was the power of the expression of the human unconscious, the underworld through which the patients were wandering. Such expression, said Philippe, summons forth *auto-curacão,* the ability of the mind to heal itself, to seize the tiller of the spirit boat and bring it forth from the shadows. The community was successful, functioning side-by-side with the more conventional treatments within the hospital. Indeed, some of Brazil's recognized artists were picked up lying comatose in the hospital's hallways and brought back to life through their own expressive powers. The institute ended with the breakdown of care for the insane in Rio, but the Casa das Palmeiras continues to exist as the largest collection of the "art of the unconscious" in the world, surely a place to go wander for a day.

Philippe first became aware of the possible efficacy of entheogens in treating mental illness when he was serving as director of the institute.

An entheogen, according to him, is a plant, such as ayahuasca or the cacti San Pedro or peyote, which brings forth the divine from within. He distinguishes them from *psychedelics*—a word meaning "mind manifesting," first coined in the early days of research with LSD—in that an entheogen is not a synthesized chemical; it has a history of human usage extending back beyond Abraham and the building of the pyramids.

"What's wrong with the word *hallucinogen*?" I asked.

"Well, etymologically, the word comes from the Latin *hallucinari,* which means 'to wander in the mind,' which is actually a pretty good description if your idea of the mind is that it encompasses more than just thinking. The word *hallucinari* has, however, taken on the meaning 'to be mistaken,' and that is not what work with daime is about."

Picking up his narrative, he related how one day a patient suffering from schizophrenia and a history of aggressive behavior came into his office. The patient had just returned from a series of treatments with some of the powerful drugs used in modern psychiatry to suppress, rather than bring catharsis to, repressed inner material.

Walking across the room, his eyes fixed on Philippe, he said over and over, "I need something stronger," ending up face-to-face with him, repeating his demand like a mantra. Feeling as though he had just been given permission to take a radical step, Philippe reached into his desk drawer and pulled out a bottle of ayahuasca. Pouring the man a cup of the acrid, brownish brew, he watched him toss it down. Instantly settling, the man left the room and began peaceably drawing, deep in concentration.

It was then that Philippe began to suspect that the entheogen might serve to gradually knit back together the fragments of the schizophrenic psyche, without causing any of the permanent damage left behind by modern drugs.

A cinnamon-colored cat with white stripes had strolled into the room and hopped into my lap as I listened to Philippe's discourse. As I stroked it, it fell asleep and began growling and scrambling its claws, struggling with an ancient enemy of its species. Waking disoriented, it stared up at me with its emerald eyes, and then went back to sleep.

Watching the interaction intently, Philippe was impressed. I didn't know why.

The music from the favela across the valley had played all night beneath the lunar glow of the monumental statue of Cristo Redentor, who soars over Rio de Janeiro like the first step up the ladder of stars.

Awaking early Christmas morning, I heard the music building into a final orgiastic intensity. Listening in groggy amazement from my bed, the partying seemed a subterfuge, a parley, an act of war. But a war against what, precisely? A conflict where the music and dance surges, until once more the seen and unseen worlds align and the dancers drop from exhaustion? Ecstasy as defense against nothingness?

I sensed that, as a northerner having crossed the equator, the lodestone I had oriented my life to had fallen away and the compass needle was swinging at random. What did purpose mean down here? What were these people fighting, what forces were arrayed against them, what did they contend against and dance with? Northern bones and abstract thought, Anglo-Saxon intention, none of it would serve when a dream-world seemed to subtly underlie my every move. What did the forces here require of me? How did one know oneself in this land?

Reaching its final, pounding crescendo, the music violently wrenched the last bit of energy from the earth, and I wondered, is to be human to be at war?

In the early evening we gathered at the Arca for the work. Men and women dressed in white freely mixed, laughing and moving with the innate elegance of the Brazilian people. Listening to the barely comprehensible sound of their Portuguese, I felt a deep, gray sadness and aloneness running like an iron bar through my chest, this strange land weighing heavily upon my senses. Before putting the cup of daime to my lips I prayed that the Arca would serve as a safe vessel for the journey on which I was about to embark.

Philippe and his partner, Mariana, took seats in front, microphones within easy reach. Musical instruments lay about. My acquaintance the cat wandered through. I sat down in a corner, next to what was to be my nemesis: the synthesizer.

People began to line up to drink. Philippe stood, carefully measuring out dosages of the brew for the participants. Fixing his gaze on me he asked, "More profound, or less profound?"

"More profound," I answered. He gave me a healthy shot. Tossing it down, I tasted the rich brown of an Amazonian river, the flavor of all the bark and leaves of the jungle. Returning to my place, I sat and waited.

The daime took its time to arrive. Songs began. A woman beckoned Philippe to her, and he performed a ritual of purification with a sword over her. I waited. After a time, we went forward to drink again.

Resuming my vigil, I suddenly felt my consciousness wheeling out of control as my isolation amplified immeasurably. Nauseous with fear, I drew each breath against hopelessness at ever escaping the agony within me. I attempted to surrender to the music but, like the creaky hinges of the doors in hell, the synthesizer beside me provided a malicious discordance, a guarantee of further suffering in a universe hopelessly out of tune.

Looking up, I saw Mariana, a sweet expression on her face, earnestly playing the accompaniment to my damnation. *I am lost,* I realized.

Have I managed to finally do it? I wondered. *Am I about to go mad in a country I don't even know? Is my psyche finally going to break from the pressures I have put upon it?* The terror of losing my soul overwhelmed me. Abandoning my meditation posture, I went to prostrate myself before the altar.

Men of the Arca were now at a row of white conga drums, pounding out an intense African rhythm. Caught up in the summons, I felt myself driven forward, the sound sweeping me out of and beyond myself. Wailing started to arise within me, coming from the deepest caverns in my psyche. The lost wail of a ghost, clinging to bushes and grasses, forever tossed among worlds.

Then it ceased. A growl rumbled low in my throat. My body strained and buckled like a chrysalis from which a new form was emerging. Suddenly, a roar was torn from my throat—a roar that devoured worlds, immaculate in its rage.

Silence. Was the silence in the room, or in my head?

My physiognomy had changed. My skull was a jaguar's.

I was a cat.

Oh shit, I thought. *Now I've really done it. I've gone and transformed into a cat in a city where nobody knows me.* I had an image of myself living on the streets of Rio, my feral eyes gleaming out from within the darkness of a cardboard box.

But then I noticed that my cat's mind was blissfully quiet. And more, the feline creature I had become felt like an old friend, an ally from beyond the sleep that rounded my little life. I felt protected and held, as if restored to some wing of my ancient phylogenetic home.

Well, either they're going to ship me back in a box and feed me raw flesh for the rest of my life, or this is just part of the journey. Either way, I concluded, *I'm not going to worry about it.*

The music really had stopped. I saw Philippe's feet before me.

"¿Roberto, estás bien?"

"¡Soy un gato!" I replied in utter bewilderment. "I'm a cat!"

Oh, Philippe shrugged, is that all? He turned around and went back to the drums.

Miração is the word used in Brazil to describe the visionary state that visits one in an ayahuasca journey. A deep miração came descending like a thick stage curtain upon me. Unable to move, I rolled over on my back as I ebbed away into distant lands. Eventually, I heard people dancing around me. Maracas were shaken over my head, summoning back my consciousness. Then a didgeridoo began its cavernous humming over my heart. Someone was holding my hand and stroking the top of my head, and I could feel my energy returning. What essential eloquence—the love and warmth of the land of the living—can be expressed through the grip of another person's hand. Then I was back. I felt my mind open from a long death.

I sat up. I was human again, and very embodied. I remembered my body, its organic unity, my hands and voice, myself. I had truly arrived in this land. But my breath was the breath of spirit.

We sat in staggered silence in a circle. The heavens had opened. Realm after realm of unimaginable subtlety and bliss, without end, poured their streaming light down upon us.

So these are the worlds beyond, I thought. *This is our birthright.*

The songs to the holy family began, rejoicing in the birth of Christ, songs beautiful beyond the reach of cathedrals. Then we danced in celebration until dawn.

Over the next couple of weeks attending the Arca, I learned that work with the daime is very centered on spirits. This was entering a new terrain, the beginnings of a whole new cartography of human experience. Sitting in the Arca, for the first time in my life, I listened to a spirit speaking through a medium. The voice in question was of a *preto velho,* one of the spirits of the dead black slaves of Brazil that are so important to the Afro-Brazilian tradition of Umbanda. The sound seemed impossible for a human voice box to fabricate: emerging as if it came from behind a curtain of water, or through dimensions of space that treated physicality like a permeable barrier.

Curiously, my mind, which had always favored its own little eccentric jaunts but whose idea of communing with the dead was to read Shakespeare or listen to the music of a Renaissance lute player after midnight, was intrigued. As if I had raised my head from the pages of the book that I thought was life, I found myself surrounded by the members of a previously unsuspected natural order. This was especially intriguing because the spirits had the same quality of objective substantiality as do all the other beings in the world.

I wished to explore other styles of work with the plant less focused on spirits, however, so when I received an invitation to join the work of another group with a strong focus on "inner work"—deep prayer with a focus on inner transformation—I accepted.

The session was called a Meditation with Grandma, and it took place in a small, quiet sanctuary in the hills far outside the roar of Rio. The "meditation" was run like a seminar: very professional, exclusive, and pricey. The group had been ongoing for years in the United States, directed by a couple that merged an orientation toward depth and transpersonal psychology with the finely honed showmanship of the traditional psychopomp, or guide of souls.

The space was open and sunny. Quartz crystals hanging in the windows sent little rainbows darting around the room, transposing the golden hope of California—the pioneer state for awakening to other forms of consciousness—to a more welcoming land. That old, persistent dream born in the '60s hasn't quite left us.

After summoning archangels for guidance and protection, a poem by a French mystic was read, which offered the self as a sacrifice to the divine, to be destroyed or exalted, however the spirit moved. And then we went forward to drink.

"Liquid sunshine," they whispered as I held the cup before me and my stomach flopped around inside like a terrified fish.

An hour later I saw, as if from a distance, that my head was bobbing drunkenly. When my head snapped upright, I was looking into a distant terrain, ancient feeling as the ruins of Pompeii, but one that I knew intimately. It was the children's shelter my mother had left me in when I was nine years old.

Without entirely losing the sensation of being an adult in that sun-filled room in Rio, I was, like one on his deathbed, plunged into my cellular memory, and the emotional and sensorial content of that land I had traveled through as a young child growing up in California. All I could do was breathe and allow this return to the place of my formation.

As she drove me to the shelter, my mother told me it would be like a summer camp from which she would come to pick me up in a month. I believed her, forming images of a Disney version of a Dickensian world where we ragged orphans would band together and have adventures, depending on one another to survive in a hostile, adult environment.

But at the front desk a cold-faced woman began rifling through my suitcase and probing the seams of my clothing for contraband. I watched her in bewilderment. Holding up my treasured Hardy Boys books, she said, "You shouldn't take these in there. The children will rip them up."

Looking at her in blank incomprehension, I wondered, *Why would someone rip up a book?*

The wail of an alarm abruptly filled the room. In my head the natural light switched to adrenaline-spiked fluorescent. "What's going on?" I asked as people hustled about behind the counter.

"The children are smoking in the bathroom again," I heard.

Children smoke?

My suitcase was returned to me. My mother gave me a hug and told me again she'd be back in a month. I drifted off in the direction she pointed, toward an open door at the far end of the room as if some gravity of fate was pulling me in. Crossing the threshold, I entered a featureless hallway, seeing only blank walls where the corridor changed direction in front of me. The walk felt endless, as if I were floating weightless between worlds.

Finally I emerged to face a table of children, all dressed in ragged T-shirts and jeans, their eyes boring into me. A man with a handlebar moustache sat at the head of the table, wearing a black leather vest that read WOLFGANG and had the slogan of a biker's club on the back. I stood frozen with my suitcase.

Wolfgang sent me to wash my hands for lunch, accompanied by a boy several years older than me. There was something in the older boy's sharply focused movements I had never seen before, and I felt that hypnotized fascination of something about to fall prey and I didn't know what to do about it.

In the tile chamber, he leaned against the wall and sized me up. "Do you smoke?" he finally asked.

This was a test, but I didn't know the right answer. His green eyes suddenly went luminous, radiant as a snake's, and my heart started to pound with fear. "No," I told him, knowing I had just failed. I returned to washing my hands.

I spent the afternoon hiding in my dorm room, but I got up the courage that evening to emerge when the girls from the adjacent wing poured in for a visit. I watched with alarm as children barely older than me climbed into one another's arms, like monkeys imitating adults. The boy with serpentine eyes, balancing a girl on his knee, turned his attention to me. Picking up a rag, he dropped it on the floor.

"Pick it up."

I walked over and handed it back to him. He dropped it on the floor again.

"Pick it up."

I looked at him, and then at all the other eyes glittering with amusement, and I burst into tears. The girl seated on his lap laughed.

I ran back into my room and slammed the door. Throwing myself on the bed, I faced the wall, still crying uncontrollably. The door opened immediately behind me, and I heard a chair being drawn up. Looking over, I saw another boy seated there with his legs crossed, another boy at his shoulder. They were a little older, and the hope flashed through my mind that they would be nice to me.

"So . . . ," the boy began, drawing out the word as he mimed holding a pad and pencil. "When did you first begin to miss your mommy?"

The boy behind him laughed sardonically. I turned back to the wall, hoping this world, like a nightmare, would go away.

The days crept by as I learned to make myself invisible in the pecking order of the place. Although the boy I shared the room with made a big deal about masturbating in the darkness (I still had no clear idea what an erection was) and claimed he pissed on my bed every night, after my initial hazing interest in me died down. One evening at dinner, after fielding a high fly ball everyone thought was a homer in an afternoon baseball game, I heard the words, "That was good catch," and I knew I was accepted.

But I still see my hands searching through the communal clothing bins, searching for the garments my mother had carefully written "Robbie" on in indelible ink, as if her handwriting could serve as a talisman to protect her son from dissolution. But they, along with my identity, had been swallowed up by the system.

One day my grandmother came to visit me. It had been three weeks, and my entire hope of salvation lay in my mother's promise to take me back home. In the visitor's cubicle my grandma sat down on the opposite side of the table and looked at me pointedly. Then she asked, "Rob, have you ever thought your mother might not come and pick you up after a month?"

I looked at her as if she were proposing the sun would not rise in the morning. "No, she said she would come at the end of a month."

"Yes, but have you considered she might not be coming?"

"No, she's going to pick me up," I said.

My grandmother winced, and stated flatly, "Robbie, you mom is not going to come at the end of the month."

I realized I was now truly an orphan, and that this had nothing to do with Disney.

One day the keepers of the prison noticed I really was a child and transferred me to the young children's ward, away from the hardened teenagers. There a pretty woman read us bedtime stories every night, trying to soothe the fresh horror of losing our mothers and fathers, to weave anew a spell of safety for us to sleep within. The nights filled with threats had come to an end, but it was too late. The place had murdered my sleep.

In my first days at the shelter I had stared at the fence of the compound, beyond which a highway roared, and conceived the idea of escape. But my nine-year-old mind floundered before the question of where I would go and what I would do. Now I was permitted to leave the jail to go to school.

As a survival technique, I taught myself how to read while walking to school, and my most vivid memories are of a deep blue sky overhead, dry heat, and the cracks and curbs of sidewalks bordered by tall, desiccated weeds. I had found *the* book, a sort of pilgrim's narrative called *The Phantom Tollbooth*. In it a boy named Milo, who also seemed to have no family, passed through a magical tollbooth and eventually ended up on a perilous quest to free the Princesses Rhyme and Reason from the Castle in the Sky where they were kept imprisoned above the Land of Ignorance. Milo's world made a lot more sense to me than the one I was living in. I began to conceive of life as a quest for some kind of meaning, but like the journey to free Rhyme and Reason, it was perilous.

Returning to the shelter from school each day I ran a gauntlet. As my feet dragged up the hill, I kept *The Phantom Tollbooth* open before me. Passing through the gates the high walls of the male juvenile hall loomed to my left. From behind the barred windows threats on my life were screamed down at me, along with demands for cigarettes or weapons. I did not look up. Then to my right I passed the yard of the female juvenile hall. Invariably the teenage girls were out that time of day, and they would all gather in the yard, pressing up against the fence, cooing about how cute I was and trying to lure me over to give them a kiss through the chain links. One day one of them clutched her arms over her jiggling breasts and, jumping up and down, cried out, "I could just squeeze you to death!"

I kept my book up and kept walking.

How long I remained gazing into the vault of the past I do not know, but eventually the miração changed course, and the pedagogical functions of ayahuasca took hold.

The universe unfolded before me as an eternal cycle of becoming and passing away, with limitless beings orbiting through countless worlds, all of it a dream. A great light and love lay in the center of this unending transmigration, I saw, the resting place that can be reached at any moment merely by remembering ourselves in it, as it. The ages weighed unimaginably heavy upon my cognition: thousands, hundreds of thousands, millions, billions of years. No end to the restless journey.

And I saw the children in the shelter in the light of this eternity. They had been my teachers. They had shown me the way to survive in the world I had fallen into, and the wounding I had sustained had been essential to that hardening, the formation of a self, capable of facing annihilation and surviving.

They, I realized with wonder, were bodhisattvas, and they had saved my life. A great love for them awoke in me, and something akin to veneration. As the worlds continued to wheel and unfold, I was carried back into another one of those deep, crystalline memories. . . .

An institution with the Maoist-sounding title of Learning House eventually took me in. An experiment in Skinnerian behavior modification, it was located next to Stanford University in Palo Alto, and it was to accustom me to living under surveillance, including by graduate students who shadowed me through the streets. Based on the tallies of our behaviors recorded during the day, we were given our behavior reinforcements for the next, which meant more privileges.

Like a board game, jargon and points ruled our lives. A PPI, or Positive Peer Interaction, earned you five hundred points and kicked you up into a more privileged sphere, as opposed to the NPI, the Negative Peer Interaction, which obviously had an opposite effect.

The behaviorist maze was benign, and blind. Asked if I would participate in a "study," I went to the university campus and sat in a lab lit by fluorescent lights and faced a bearded, long-boned graduate student. Setting his contraption before me like an earnest young Jesuit with a sacred machine, he handed me a remote control wrapped in black electrical tape.

I studied it, and then the machine: a miniature stage covered with sharp, cold, metallic objects like barbed wire, tacks, and Brillo pads. "Press the button," he said.

I did and the stage rotated to reveal an artfully arranged pile of sweets: cookies, chocolates, candies.

What the hell?

My job, I learned, was to simply sit before the device, concentrating my attention on the contents of the stage, and then after a few minutes I could press the button and concentrate on its opposite. So we began. I pressed the button and stared. The young doctor observed. The fluorescents burned. The minutes stretched and wobbled. The cold pile ate its own tail and the warm pile drifted away and disintegrated into the air.

Finally, the young doctor broke the silence, saying, "That's enough for now. Thank you for your participation, Robbie." I relaxed.

Leaning back in his chair, he said in an offhand way, "You can eat the cookies, if you want." All of his careful thesis design, all the scrutinizing of the committee for research on human subjects, all of his professor's advice, hung on that moment. Had I been deconditioned from my natural boyish appetite for cookies?

"No, thanks," I said. But they forgot I was not a rat. Having passed through the world of internments, I refused gifts because I no longer trusted the giver. My conditioning was far deeper than he ever imagined.

My strange year-and-a-half-long odyssey ended when my father attempted to introduce me to his suburban life. My stint in the child prisons was never spoken of, but I already saw myself as a black sheep.

The incarceration had torn the fabric of my belonging to society, and despite my best efforts to be a good boy and forget, nothing could knit back up that hole in my soul. As the years of elementary school and junior high school passed, I began quietly calibrating the evidence that the society around me, my father's world, was a lie.

The bubble burst one day when my best friend Gordon returned from England with an album called *Never Mind the Bollocks, Here's the Sex Pistols*. Johnny Rotten's raging voice seared our minds. The music was an explosion of inchoate energy, the lyrics a nihilistic apocalypse. Punk rock offered salvation through anger, and since I was slowly dying in an existential vacuum anyway, why not give that dying some significance?

By the time I was fourteen I knew who the enemy was, marching in their long plastic lines of death. It was the men in suits, the automatons following the rules, the believers waving flags.

It was better to die than lose your soul believing in the world they had created. So one night I packed a change of clothes and, clutching my record albums in a bundle, jumped out the window and ran off like a hunted animal through the high grasses surrounding our suburban development. Now a refugee, I began wandering the streets, from one scene to another.

Finally, in my fifteenth year, a man in a suit got me. Walking through downtown Fairfield I saw a flight of stairs leading to a roof. Climbing up, I sat looking down on the street below and started to roll a joint but, before I could finish, an apparition appeared. A blue suit, red tie, and florid red nose topped by white hair was coming forward to seize me. Quickly stuffing the marijuana back into my pocket, I turned to face the apparition of the enemy who demanded to look into my backpack.

"No way, man. I know my rights," I retorted, and walked down the stairs and around the corner, and then broke into a run. After a few blocks I stopped, thinking, *Whew, wasn't that strange!*

Police cars came to a screeching halt in a circle around me, and guns were leveled at me from behind their hoods. I raised my hands in the air in a litany that was to become excruciatingly predictable with time. But then it was new. I was searched, my bag of shake found, the contents of my backpack rifled through, and I went to prison.

A month passed in a cell in Solano County Juvenile Hall, a month of empty threats and collective herding. Finally I was told I was going to see a judge, and myself and several other ragged children were led through a tunnel and made to sit in an antechamber of concrete, where we idly read the graffiti.

Above, the forces of justice were assembled, including my own public defender, a smart young man wearing John Lennon glasses. Eventually I emerged from the underground world of concrete and bars into a plush courtroom with upholstered seats, polished wood, carpets, and suits.

I saw my father sitting in the spectators' gallery. He wouldn't look at me.

Welcoming me, my lawyer told me to relax. I asked who the prosecutor was, and he pointed out a young woman in a suit. I thought, *Great. A woman will have some compassion.* The blue suit and red tie was there. He was a jeweler, and I had inadvertently walked upon the roof of his shop, summoning up his own fearful apparitions of robbers drilling in through the ceiling. When asked to identify me, he did so gladly, but added I had long hair at the time of my trespassing. Like me, he had seen what he had most feared and despised: I had not had a haircut since my incarneration.

Then the young woman in the suit argued that although my offense was mild this time, I was clearly on the way to becoming a dangerous criminal and I should be sent to prison while there was still time. I knew what that meant: CYA, the California Youth Authority. Word leaked out from that place. It was San Quentin for kids.

Swinging in panic to my defender, he patted my arm and told me it was going to be okay. I looked back at this avenging fury of Solano County, who studiously avoided my eyes.

My defender spoke briefly, to the point. The judge told them to let me go and dropped the misdemeanor charges of trespassing and possession. Filled by a flood of relief, I turned to my father, but, still refusing to look at me, he rose and, clearing his throat, asked permission to address the court.

"My son is out of control, and needs to be restrained," he began. "He needs to be kept in a secure facility. . . . " I realized he was asking them to lock me back up. As I sat listening to my father request my destruction, my soul recoiled even further back into the depths I had just barely emerged from.

The judge was having none of it. He was a big man, and in his robe he was imposing. He explained that his decisions were final and my father was acting inappropriately. My father sat down. I was free to wander through the system, of incarcerations and group homes, foster homes, crash pads, and the street.

Leaning into the miração, waves of light breaking through my mind, I suddenly saw everything through the eyes of my father. My perspective was no longer that of a wounded raging boy, it was that of a man raised in a deeply conservative world, cherishing certain assumptions about society and human development, believing in his own goodness as much as I did in my own.

My mind grasped the parameters of his perspective: naïve belief in the system, the supreme value of control, and shame at failing his son. I saw he could have acted in no other way. His request I be sent to prison was his expression of love for me.

The furnaces at Auschwitz, the massacres committed by the Crusaders at Jerusalem, the tortures of the Inquisition—all flowed past me, and drunk with the soothsaying vine, I saw that their fundament is love.

But this wasn't the love of smiling cherubim, or even light-streaming saviors. This love was geologic, like plate tectonics, subducting us like the fragile memories of fossils into its superheated core. It was elemental, birthing us and the constellations in each moment, and consuming us utterly in the next. Before this love, what is the ignorance of humans? All our actions arise from, and their trajectories ultimately dissolve into, this boundless love of the Creator. As do we.

If we choose to remember.

Otherwise, the apple's toxin that gave us the illusion of separate identity allows us to wander in the revolving worlds for multiple eternities.

The work was done. My recoil into the depths of disillusion, at my father's words years before, released. My father loved me.

Sitting on the loo with my pants around my ankles, I had plumbed the ancient theological paradox of theodicy: How can evil exist in a universe whose creator is love?

Like the *finis* marking the end of a book, I flushed the toilet. Fastening my belt, I stood and opened the door. The room was in deep silence, the participants motionless, concentrated. Light spilled everywhere. Walking to the sink as if I was taking my first steps on earth, I opened the spigot. Water gushed forth as spirit.

Stirring the deep silence in the room, I involuntarily said, "Thank you God," and began to wash my hands, and then continued on to my face, baptizing myself in this new realization.

I dried off and went to sit down, but my body was exuberant, celebratory, alive again. I asked permission to do some movements, and as the energy began flowing through my body, a flute suddenly sounded behind me. The shaman had quietly come up and was playing an Arabic melody, sinuous and irresistible, and I danced until I had expressed my joy at my true release from prison.

Philippe welcomed me on my return, curious about how my work had gone with the other group. I gave him a sketch, joining him on his patio overlooking Rio for a coffee.

Philippe nodded. The fundamental principle of work with entheogens, he told me as I sat, dazed and happy in the morning light, is autocuração. Drugs impose upon or suppress states and conditions in the body and mind, but they rarely reach to those depths within our own being that are capable of orchestrating our own healing.

According to Philippe, all too often drugs merely mask human suffering. Plant medicines, on the other hand, possess an intelligence of their own, are allies, and work their way, like brilliantly colored serpents, as far as the twinings of our DNA. In short, medicines, as gifts of nature, possess intelligence that drugs, manufactured by humans, do not.

But pragmatically, I wondered, what differences are there between drugs and medicines? For a drug-ridden society like the United States—whether we're talking crack scored off a dealer on the street or Prozac pushed by the pharmaceutical giants—what do these native medicines have to offer us that we don't already enjoy with our chemicals?

Philippe raised his hand and spread his fingers before me.

"Five!" he said.

"Five what?"

"Five fundamental differences between chemicals and plants," he said, as if revealing a mystical theorem underlying the superficial appearances of reality. He went on to explain them in depth.

The first is the pedagogical nature of the experience. With entheogens, there is a phenomenon of an inner voice, a voice coming from outside the boundaries of the ego, which, from its far greater perspective, balances the self. This sage voice instructs and corrects, gives insight, reveals ways. Philippe gave the example of the many individuals in the churches of Daime in Brazil who have no formal education, yet display the theological sophistication of graduates from divinity schools.

A second difference is the religious and ethical nature of the experience. Medicinal plants bring about a confrontation with the shadow contents of the psyche, revealing "sin" and often triggering public confession of crimes, however petty. The purgative dimension to this experience (it is not unusual for such cleansing to trigger vomiting) suggests that sin—behavior stemming from greed, hatred, or ignorance that harms the self and/or others—occupies the body as well as the psyche, and has to be purged from the organism like any other disease. While this cleansing of the conscience is often harrowing, it leaves a deep sense of repentance, absolution, and new opportunity in its wake. All too often, drugs intervene in or mask suffering, but they cannot effect transformation at the root of suffering.

The third is the medicines' therapeutic properties. Effective in treating depression, aggressiveness, and addiction, they also help with emotional catharsis, ease physical suffering, and can bring about physical cures, including for a disease such as cancer.

"Cancer?" I interrupted, my pen hovering over the dread word. "Ayahuasca can heal cancer?"

"When administered in the proper setting by a skilled healer, oh yes," Philippe replied. I was so high I could believe just about anything at that moment, but *that* one I would have to see for myself, I decided.

Ironically, Philippe continued, while the drugs normally prescribed to treat such conditions can cause irreversible damage to the organism, the much-feared entheogens, *when used with experienced guides in a ritual context,* are completely safe. Pregnant women drink daime in Brazil. I met a woman in my subsequent journey to the Brazilian state of Acre who drank each time she gave birth, and her three children are beautiful, flourishing young people. Entheogens also may aid in healing psychotic breaks and schizophrenia, gradually knitting the psyche back together because their therapeutic properties are multidimensional, working physically, mentally, and spiritually.

A fourth feature of entheogens is the occurrence of paranormal experience in conjunction with their usage. Precognition and telepathy are common. Synchronistic events multiply. One delightful example is "Indian movies," or Cinema de Indio. When a member of a tribe in the Amazon wants to know how his family member or friend is doing at some distant geographical point, he drinks some ayahuasca and enters into his friend's experience, and then comes back with the news. Such claims are naturally controversial, but healers such as María Sabina have spontaneously demonstrated this capacity to researchers.

Finally, entheogens facilitate the development of the psyche. In the churches of Daime, the children in Brazil who drink ayahuasca suffer little from hyperactivity, aggressiveness, or difficulty with concentrated thought. An overall development of consciousness, awareness of God, and the interconnectivity of all life, along with a deeper maturation of the psyche, appear to occur in individuals who take entheogens as a sacrament over a long period of time.

Interestingly enough, Philippe's five principles have been confirmed by numerous studies. According to Susana Bustos, researchers such as Grob have "found that regular and long-term participation in ayahuasca rituals in a Brazilian religious context decreases self-destructive behavior, including addiction, while it increases general psychological maturity, socially sensitive behavior, and healthy abilities to cope with life."[1] Other researchers such as Silveira have "found similar results in Brazilian adolescents belonging to the Santo Daime and UDV cults, including radical changes in value-systems toward others and oneself, as well as significantly higher scores on some neuropsychological capacities compared to the control group."[2] Gimaraes Dos Santos and Santos et al. also "report decreased psychometric measures of anxiety, panic-like symptoms, and hopelessness in experienced Daime practitioners under acute effects of ayahuasca."[3] And finally, on the medical side, "positive healing effects of the ritual use of ayahuasca on cancer have been shown" by researchers such as Quinlan and Topping.[4]

After my conversation with Philippe I made a little journey through the pulsing streets of Rio in the gritty afternoon sunshine. Returning to sit in the café whose awning had once faded into a forest canopy, it now felt solider, more firmly incarnated. Keeping an eye out for the man with the elegant soliloquies, I reviewed my notes of the previous couple of weeks spent in what was turning into a land of miracles. Even though the potent effects of the vine had worn off, the joy and lightness in my body and spirit remained. It felt as if I had drunk the generative power of nature itself.

I realized that Philippe's theories about ayahuasca's "pedagogical nature" fit my experience like a glove. A sage voice, coming from far outside the boundaries of my ego, had reinterpreted my traumatic childhood for me, showing it to me from a vastly more mature perspective. I felt the terrible burden of self-annihilation I had carried for decades within myself lightened. I was given a new opportunity in life, indeed, the beginnings of a new childhood to live from.

And it had shown me the way of forgiveness with my father. In seeing beyond my own wounded, raging perspectives, I was finally absolved from the internal guilt of having borne him such anger for so long.

The plant, in short, had taken me through a catharsis and a spiritual awakening that decades of therapy, churchgoing, or meditation might have never achieved. Yet I had to travel to Brazil to experience the extraordinary therapeutic and spiritual potentials of this plant.

In the United States, ayahuasca has received little serious study in the medical and psychiatric communities at large. In fact, because ayahuasca contains DMT, it is formally *illegal* to study it (unless you're capable of leaping through the endless hoops imposed by the FDA), much less heal oneself with it.*

Strangely enough, by virtue of gathering in a sacred enclosure to work with entheogens, I had joined a long lineage of mystics, witches, and alchemists—the shamans of the West—and could now be imprisoned by a culture still terrified by having eaten an apple and awoken in abrupt exile from the Garden.

---

*There are signs of change in the air, however. In a surprise move, the United States Supreme Court ruled unanimously on February 21, 2006, that a North American branch of the Brazilian ayahuasca church União do Vegetal (UDV), located in New Mexico, can continue using their sacrament as part of their regular religious ceremonies—at least for the time being. The legal struggle began in 1999 when federal drug agents raided the Santa Fe home of UDV leader Jeffrey Bronfman and confiscated thirty gallons of the UDV's ayahuasca. The UDV sued the government on the grounds that their use of *hoasca* (their term for the plant medicine) is central to their religious beliefs and practices and should be protected under the 1990 Religious Freedom Restoration Act (RFRA). But there is a caveat to the Supreme Court ruling: the decision in this case, known officially as *Gonzales v. O Centro Espírita Beneficiente União do Vegetal,* does not legalize ayahuasca. It merely affirms a preliminary injunction previously requested by the UDV to stop the Drug Enforcement Agency from confiscating UDV hoasca and arresting church members until the conclusion of a U.S. district court trial. That trial, still not begun as of this writing, will examine the religious freedom issues involved in much greater depth.[5]

Recalling my harrowing transformation into a jaguar, it occurred to me that renouncing the placebo knowledge of exile for the sake of real experience of the Garden leads to the discovery of unusual ancestors—some wearing face paint and feathers, others sequestered with retorts and alembics, some coated with fur and walking about on all fours.

Man, this is potent stuff, I thought, setting down my coffee. If approached and studied with reverence instead of fear, couldn't this medicine that had been discovered by the indigenous tribes of the Amazon bring about a revolution in the science of Western medicine and psychology?

3 Fear No Spirits

Horatio: Oh day and night, but this is
wondrous strange!
Hamlet: And therefore as a stranger give
it welcome.

SHAKESPEARE, *HAMLET*

Acre is the holy land for work with daime in Brazil. Bordering Peru and Bolivia, it is the westernmost state of the Amazon basin, and it still possesses 90 percent of its original forest. Acre is very much raw frontier, hosting some of the heaviest cocaine trafficking in South America, a powerful presence of evangelical Christianity, and serious rural poverty. It was also the home state of Chico Méndes, who, in resistance to the massive land theft and senseless deforestation being practiced by the wealthy newcomers to Acre in the 1980s, organized and imbued the forest workers of the Amazon with an environmental vision. This was a fight that Méndes continued up to the day of his murder by a local rancher and strongman.

Philippe and other members of the Arca had sent me onward in my pilgrimage to the small city of Rio Branco in Acre, over two thousand miles away, to experience the roots of the daime movement in Brazil. Joining me in this journey was my friend Sean, a botanist and tree-climbing instructor who had shown up in Rio with a Wyatt Earp mustache and tales of wild Brazilian women. After participating in a couple of ceremonies at the Arca, Sean decided to accompany me.

"They're going to learn about discipline there," Philippe had said, laughing. My stomach tightened with apprehension. What if I underwent another transformation into a jaguar smack in the middle of a ceremony?

Within the movement that had begun with Mestre Irineu, two main streams had developed: the Church of the Universal Flowing Light, or Santo Daime, which claims to hold most truly to the original form transmitted by the Mestre; and the Barquinha, or "little boat," whose work, with marked Afro-Brazilian elements, was initiated by a disciple of Irineu's, Daniel Pereira de Mattos (known as Frei Daniel). As well, there are the native traditions underlying the lineage of Mestre Irineu, as practiced for thousands of years by the indigenous peoples of the Amazon basin. Arising and co-evolving out of the people's seamless communion with the forest, these traditions emerge from the womb and gift of Pachamama, the Quechua name for the Earth Mother.

Although we didn't know this at the time, seeds of distrust toward foreigners had been sown throughout the communities. Among the Indians, biopiracy by Westerners, who ingratiate themselves into local tribes and smuggle out their healing plants only to patent them and reap profits for themselves (sending back baseball caps and T-shirts by way of compensation), have alienated the healers of the forest. Some tribes and healers, therefore, have begun keeping their medicines to themselves.

The extent of this tragedy cannot be fully appreciated until our dependence on indigenous medicinal knowledge is fully acknowledged. After all, as anthropologist Jeremy Narby writes, "74 percent of the modern pharmacopoeia's plant-based remedies were first discovered by 'traditional' societies; to this day, less than 2 percent of all plant species have been fully tested in laboratories, and the great majority of the remaining

98 percent are in the tropical rainforests. . . . The biodiversity of tropical forests [represents] a fabulous source of unexploited wealth, but without the botanical knowledge of indigenous people, biotechnicians would be reduced to testing blindly the medicinal properties of the world's estimated 250,000 plant species."[1] The folly of alienating native healers, or allowing them to go extinct, is further underlined by ethnobotanist Mark Plotkin, who witnessed a traditional healer curing severe type 2 diabetes with a preparation of plants (their healing efficacy turned out to be nonreplicable in the laboratory). He notes that "contrary to what many believe, for the foreseeable future, *the value of nature as a source of novel compounds with therapeutic applications increases (rather than diminishes) as technology advances.*"[2]

As well, certain Daime communities have closed their doors to participation by Westerners after receiving what they perceived to be bad press. Many also will no longer donate bottles of ayahuasca to foreign visitors after seeing the sacrament smuggled into the United States and sold at a profit.

In spite of these abuses, we found the doors of most churches open to us; the pilgrim is welcome to join in the ceremonies, which they call simply *um trabalho:* "a work."

Struggling with our bags and attempting to orient ourselves after the three-day bus ride from Rio de Janeiro to Rio Branco, Sean and I encountered Luis, a young lawyer from São Paulo who had recently transplanted himself to Rio Branco to work on environmental issues and indigenous rights. Fortunately for us, he spoke a pidgin English that he had learned from his mother. Small of stature, clean-cut, and alert, he seemed to engage the world around him with a boundless optimism. It turned out he was a daimista, a member of a Barquinha church. He offered his assistance, as well as his opinions about the communities we had come to visit. This gave me some pause. The usual rivalries among groups existed in Rio Branco too, I decided.

That afternoon he met us at our hotel and oriented us to the work of the Barquinhas, explaining that the church of the "little boat" is a synthesis of Catholic Christianity and Umbanda and Candomble, the Yoruba spiritual practices brought over by the slaves from Africa. He elucidated a very complicated system of correspondences among deities: Oxala, the masculine father spirit, related to Christ; Yemanja, the Holy Mother, feminine power, related to Mary; other Orixas, or spirits, such as Oxossi, related to the power of the forest and native healing wisdom; and Xango, the power of justice, related to stones and through his spouse, Oxum, to waterfalls. I scrambled to take notes, despairing of distinguishing mantra from yantra from tantra.

No matter. We were going to get to experience Umbanda. The community was in the midst of a twenty-day-long *romería,* a cycle of worship of São Sebastião (Saint Sebastian) in which they drank ayahuasca every night, and there was to be a major work soon.

But the first visit of my pilgrimage was, fittingly, to Alto Santo. Leaving Sean at a little party we had gotten drawn into in the hotel's restaurant, I took a bus to one of the first churches founded by Irineu Serra located thirty minutes outside of Rio Branco close to the site of the Mestre's mausoleum. The bus rumbled there in the night, upon dirt roads through an area that still felt carved out of the jungle. It was warm, the stars were bright, and the slat-board pioneer houses I passed were dark.

Descending from the bus, I walked down a road filled with humming insects and, upon turning a corner, a vision leaped electric, out of the darkness. Beneath blazing fluorescent lights, I saw two lines of men and women dancing, facing one another beneath a huge, open-air structure. A gigantic cross with two crossbeams (the Caravaca Cross adopted from northern Spain, the second crossbeam representing the second coming of Christ), stood illuminated in the front yard.

Music and singing arose from the structure—a sound like a polka band playing in the back of a flatbed truck on their way to heaven. As I drew closer I saw the women wore white dresses with green sashes, multicolored ribbons descending from their shoulders. The men wore white suits with a green pinstripe descending their pant legs. Entering, dazzled by the lights and colors, I saw that the men also wore a silver brooch in the shape of a Star of David with a crescent moon resting within, indicating they were *fardados*.*

The women were wearing silver crowns. They were doing a four-step dance, moving back and forth in a tightly disciplined line, beating out their steps with maracas. In the center was a band, jamming on accordion, conga drum, tambourine, electric guitar, bass, and classical guitar. The high pitch of the women's voices over it all gave me the image of a psychedelic subway train charging, relentless and happy, through the night.

I was welcomed and, in a numinous daze, I was led across the concrete floor to a booth at the far end of the structure, where a dignified man with a bushy moustache waited like an amiable bartender. Looking within the booth, I saw an altar. A candle sat upon it, burning before an antique photo of a stocky forest worker, his expression transported, gazing into another world. The altar was covered with huge bottles of ayahuasca.

Smiling at me, the daimisita poured, waiting for my signal to stop. I drank and a seat was set out for me. I sat and tried to follow the hymns of the dancers, but the Portuguese was very fast. Someone next to me handed me a hymnal. I closed my eyes and listened; angelic mists and swirling mandalas began to draw me on.

I opened my eyes. The music had stopped. I saw a new frontier, a new people without artifice, a world of exquisite possibilities. This, I realized, is the new frontier for humanity, open and immeasurably happy.

My language acquisition abilities had somehow been radically enhanced, and I could understand the Portuguese being spoken around me. Entering into conversation with Henrique, a professor of mathematics and physics at the University of Acre, I discussed with him the Buddhist doctrine of *sunyata,* emptiness, and its relation to work with entheogens. Henrique began asking me penetrating questions about the United States, which stirred an immense well of sadness within me. The

---

Fardado is sometimes translated as "star person"—giving a New Age airiness to a fundamentally military conception: *farda* in Portuguese describes a "military uniform."

face of my beloved homeland was changing irrevocably and I could not speak for grief. Henrique looked at me with comprehension.

"The daime is working on you, isn't it?" he asked.

As the music commenced again, I took a maraca and joined the line, getting down the four-step but giving up on my attempts to sing from the hymnal at the same time. Later I was taken to the altar and introduced to the figure in the photo: it was Mestre Raimundo Irineu Serra. I studied him. He looked as if he were wearing a Noh mask, the one that represented vision into other worlds. I made my bows. May the humble inherit the earth. It appeared to be happening right there.

Sean was a good traveling partner who possessed an instinctual gentility. A musician, he kept a guitar slung over his shoulder and you could almost see his tail wagging as he set off down the street to find a nightclub. He also suffered fools gladly, having an affinity with the three basic instincts of Brazilian life: *cachaça, mulheres,* and *samba,* that is to say, wine, women, and song.

The following morning in our hotel, he came up to my room ready to set out for some breakfast. I was still contemplating my evening at Alto Santo. Cracking open the heavy shutters over my window, I swung them open and found myself face to face with three smiling Brazilians, who all gave me the thumbs up sign.

"They've been waiting for you, Robert," he laughed, clapping me on the shoulder.

"What happened to your mustache?"

"Oh, well, you remember that girl who was playing guitar in the restaurant last night before you left?"

"Yeah."

"Well, she named me Tex, and whenever she saw me she would make her hands into pistols and draw them from her hips and go, pow pow! I got sick of it."

"Kind of cute though, huh?"

"She wasn't my type," he stated flatly. "But have you seen the owner of this hotel, man? You're not going to believe this, but she knows we're here to do ayahuasca."

"I know. When I was sitting in the restaurant she asked me if I was a member of the Santo Daime. I thought there must be some secret society operating here. I laughed and told her if I was, I wasn't aware of it."

"She saw us talking with Luis."

"Small town, huh?"

"How was the ceremony?"

I gave him an account, imitating the dance with a "boom chucka chucka boom chucka chucka."

"Okay," he said. "I'm ready to go to the Barquinha church tonight. Let's get some breakfast and go check out the town."

Rio Branco, we discovered that day, is a riparian town bordering both sides of a wide, slow-moving river of the same name. From the river's edge, where funky warrens of markets stand on stilts over riverbanks littered with plastic, the town extends into a commercial center. Wide parks filled with stands selling the fruits of the jungle, hammocks, and local crafts are bordered by fortresslike government buildings and eateries catering to the Brazilian appetite for rain forest beef.

The heat is thick and the inhabitants tend to stick to the shade during the days. Afternoons are punctuated by torrential showers coming out of the surrounding jungle and then disappearing back into it again. Besides the graceful old trees in the park and the movement of goods harvested from the jungle, there is little presence of the teeming wild lying outside Rio Branco's borders. In the night the town comes to life, when groups of *capoeiristas* gather in circles to practice their acrobatic martial art on the street corners to the thrumming of the African bowed instrument, the *berimbaus*. Nightclubs pulse with the music of *forro*, the tight and sexy dance loved by Brazilians.

Outside the concrete center of the town, Acre hosts a landscape dotted with churches of Daime, which light up at night like phosphorescent jellyfish floating in a dark, tropical sea.

The Barquinhas wear sailor's suits when they make a major journey, bright white with epaulettes and a white cap like a fez with a braid wound around it. They are right to do so. During the ceremony I saw my guardian angel, my guiding spirit, as a blazing figurehead on the prow of the ship of my soul, cutting through the darkness with his omniscience, and I realized the carven prows of those old Viking ships were no mere decorations.

Arriving at the Barquinha church in the company of Luis a couple of evenings after my visit to Alto Santo, Sean and I passed through a wooden gate and entered an open structure like the one where people danced in Alto Santo, except the floor was of hard-packed, red earth. In the center, spread out on a surface of sand, I noticed miniature figures arranged in a village scene. Continuing down a flight of stairs, we entered the patio of the church, a cross lit up at the entryway, a dirty little scamp of a dog curled up right on the threshold. It could be any Catholic church in Latin America, with its bell tower and niches for saints, its exterior a muted orange painted over smooth adobe.

We and everyone else stepped over the dog, respecting its presence there, and entered. Within, we crossed a clean floor of white tile and faced an altar covered with images of saints. A massive banquet table with a white tablecloth surrounded by chairs sat in the middle of the room. A statue of São Sebastião, chained to a tree and pierced by arrows, sat upon the table. Rows of seats lined the back and both sides of the church.

I wandered off and sat on the wrong side. A musician tuning his guitar gestured me back: women sat on one side, men on the other. Looking around, I noted that most of the faces were of African descent, unlike in the Santo Daime church in Alto Santo.

Luis left us, and Sean and I sat quietly in the pews. Finally a bell rang, and Luis reappeared dressed in white and gestured for us to come. We went out and saw two lines had formed, one of women and the other of men, and they were filing forward to drink ayahuasca. Once we reached the head of the line, we were given the sacrament. We made the sign of the cross with the cup, and drank. The ayahuasca was very bitter and strong.

We went back in and took our seats. The core of the community took their places around the banquet table. A curtain had been drawn over the altar, covering the entire front of the church. The mantric cycle of praise commenced, most of which I didn't understand, except I could recognize the Credo being repeated over and over, and the names of Jesus, Mary, the Heavenly Father, and São Sebastião. Musicians accompanied the prayer.

As the ayahuasca began to take hold, I noticed the curtains were slowly parting in front of the altar. I heard a voice say to me, "Fear no spirits." *Okay,* I thought, *I don't fear spirits.* In fact, I suddenly felt completely comfortable with them.

Something very powerful began moving, like a spiritual storm front, through the church. People rose from their seats and stood, very erect, two fingers of their right hand raised at the level of their faces like antennae. Piercing whistling tore through the air, sounds I cannot imagine the human vocal apparatus capable of making.

The spirits of the *preto velhos,* the old blacks, had come, and the group possessed by the African spirits filed out.

Luis reappeared beside us, smiling. "Time to drink again," said our happy maitre d'. I looked out and sure enough, the line was forming anew. Sean and I looked at each other in disbelief. I started to say, "I think I may actually have had enough already . . . ," but then I shrugged and we went out and drank.

The curtain was parting more rapidly now, in imitation of the opening of the heavenly realm, and then the ayahuasca struck like a blinding cloud of light. Seated in profound miração I beheld the blazing guardian of my spirit boat, as an intricate ritual of prostration was carried out by men and women in sailor's suits facing the altar before me. In the middle of a song I came to Christ and laid my burden down before him, my long journey filled with wounds and bewilderment. I felt his hand on my forehead and I saw the shell of my former self in California and felt deep compassion for the lonely man I had been.

It all seemed a blaze of light, a stupefaction, a vanishing, the guitar and Catholic liturgy weaving fresh neural pathways through my mind.

The curtains slowly closed, and the community vanished to doff their sailor suits. Luis reappeared and announced, "The evening is just beginning."

Sean and I looked at each other in astonishment. How could we take any more? We already felt irradiated by spirit. But the lines to drink were forming again outside. "We're moving on into the tantra, the Umbanda portion of the work now," Luis explained.

Going out to the structure with its floor of packed red earth, I had an opportunity to study the figures arranged in the sand in the center. Luis explained they were the Holy Family, or rather, the Holy Ancestors, the Yorimba. Their skin was deeply black, their garments and eyes pearly white, and they were spread out in a tableau of village life. One fellow played the banjo; the white-haired, ample matriarch was enthroned in the center; the patriarch, thin and tall like a reed and capable of walking a hundred miles at a stretch through arid ground, stood beside her. At their backs, as if on the other side of the world, was the European Holy Family, little white-skinned baby Jesus in his cradle, Joseph and Mary and a donkey in attendance, angels guarding the way.

The band commenced, conga drums prominent. Luis turned to me and said, "Whatever you do, don't stop dancing." It was a slow dance, widdershins, men and women moving in two circles, a dance to draw energy and life out of the earth.

I began awkwardly, but eventually got the hang of it: a four-step inside a square, and then a step forward. In the center, many women and a few men were smoking pipes, using the tobacco for purification and to send messages to the divinity, spitting and bowing, hunched over close to the earth. After a time I saw Luis, his arms folded behind his back, pipe in mouth, stooped forward in a posture of aged dignity close to the altar. Somehow he made me think of a young Abe Lincoln. Young women were led around and in by their elders, and the sick and simple were brought forward. The earth became wet with spit. The drums beat. We moved in a circle around the center, but the center did not radiate out. Rather it absorbed our energy. It was dark, inchoate, liminal. A *bardo* space, the votive pit in Hades in which Odysseus spilled the blood of the ewe and ram, and poured libations to summon the unnumbered dead . . . a terminal where the spirits negotiate their transit to other worlds.

The power went out, and candles were lit, blazing, scintillating around the forms of the dancers in white. It was breathtakingly beautiful, and I began to understand the dance: the power of old Africans, pulse rising from the earth, ayahuasca working through body. I was grateful to be allowed to dance on the periphery and not get drawn in. I did fear those spirits. I was not ready to experience *atuação,* or mediumship, with the spirits of Umbanda.

An old man was dancing out there in the crowd—a mulatto, stringy from a life of hard work, dirt poor. Sean had taken a seat and I walked over and clapped him on the back. We were both smiling in rapture.

"See that old man?" Sean asked me, tipping his head in the old forest worker's direction.

"Yep. He's been checking us out."

"I want to be an old man like him, drinking ayahuasca and dancing with the spirits."

We decided we loved this old man.

The old man came around in the circle of dancers again and we watched him. He pretended not to be observing us, but I smiled and gave him the thumbs-up sign. Breaking into a huge grin, he nodded back at us. He must have loved us too.

The dance concluded in the dark of the early morning. As Sean and I rode back together in a taxi, he turned to me from the front seat and said, "Man, I don't know how I am going to return to my life in California after this."

My own life there seemed so inconceivably distant, I could only nod in agreement. My Western intellect, which I had imagined as fairly open, had had all its fundamental premises blown that evening. The only useful shred of the Western intellectual tradition I could think of was, "There are more things in Heaven and Earth, Horatio, than are dreamt of in our philosophy."

Luis and I had arranged to meet in the center of Rio Branco, not far from where I had stood earlier in the day watching children leap from the girders of the bridge into the brown swirling waters of the river fifty feet below. A smell of burning plastic wafted through the marketplace, but bars selling pitchers of juice from the cornucopia of fruit growing in the Amazon compensated for the stench.

It was a couple days later, and Sean had been pretty much shut up in his hotel room since the night at the Barquinha, playing guitar and watching Brazilian television. I was out and about, but had the same problem as he: What does one do with one's life after having gone to the heavenly realms? The world seemed dull and gray in comparison.

That evening was solely a work of mantra, of praise, and while I still didn't know what to make of tantra, I had a deep feeling of gratitude for my experience of it. Luis appeared and while we waited for a local bus to take us to the Barquinha church, a young man, his hair and beard gone wild, came ranting through the station, a voice crying from the wilderness, and a sign of the strength of the evangelical movement in Acre. The Brazilians didn't seem to do anything halfway in this land of spirits.

The bus came and we boarded. Talking about the situations in Brazil that seemed especially designed to push a North American's buttons, I hazarded the opinion that sometimes anger can help set things straight.

Luis turned and looked me in the eyes. "There is never any reason to get angry. Ever."

I looked back and realized he was right. Fierce defense in preservation of the world is one thing. Anger at a person or situation is another. North Americans, I realized, have an illusion of a right to elbow room that Brazilians know doesn't exist. In fact, we even accept anger as a kind of social lubricant. I fell silent.

Changing the subject, he explained to me that when the preto velhos came that evening and entered the bodies and minds of the mediums of the church, I could go for an interview with one of them. He would translate for me. I would need him because the old Africans speak with very thick, archaic accents.

Later that evening a little girl came and tapped my thigh while I sat in the church, gesturing for me to follow. I entered a back room with another floor of hard packed red earth. Those who had been possessed by the preto velhos earlier in the evening had taken up their places within, lined up against the walls in their consultories, altars of African and Christian figures by their sides, pipes smoking. It was a scene transported straight from Africa.

Luis met me at the door and led me up to a small black woman with a grave but pleasant expression, sitting close to the earth on a stool, a pipe in her hand. She was not old, but somehow she gave the impression of being wizened. Taking another stool, I sat before her. I was told I could ask her any question, or if I have an illness she can work on it. Anything I wanted.

Gulping down my shame, I asked the classic phone psychic question. "Grandmother, when am I going to find my partner? A woman that can share my life's work with me? I am almost forty and I still haven't found her. . . ."

Stammering to a halt, I fell silent, asking myself, *Did I have to travel all the way to the jungles of Brazil to ask something so naive?*

But the young/old woman's eyes narrowed in her head. Leaning forward on her stool, she replied in a rhythmical Portuguese that utterly eluded me. Luis translated. "You will certainly meet her, there is no doubt. But you need to relax. It will take longer for her to appear if you are tense."

She added it would help if I lit a candle to my guardian spirit and took a shower with certain herbs. I relaxed. Whoever these old Africans may be, they were thoroughly down to earth.

Not to mention dead-on accurate, I was soon to discover.

Emboldened, I asked a second question.

"Grandmother, I keep encountering a cat, a black panther. Who is this creature, and what is my relationship to it?"

"All people have an animal," she said, her expression suggesting the answer to my question was a bit obvious. "The cat is a powerful protector, and very loving. But she also has a dark side. The claws and teeth of the black panther know no limits. She would consume the world in her rage."

"Open your hands," she told me.

She stood and put her palms on mine, and then she lightly feathered my forehead, saying prayers over me. She sat back down and regarded me shrewdly. I thanked her. I told her I was very happy to be there.

"You are very welcome to our church," she replied.

Luis, who had been translating, added, "I think they like you."

I made a short bow and went out.

The romería finished for the evening, but the daime was not done with me. Standing outside trying to speak I found my eyes closing and my consciousness drifting off. My interlocutor, a tall, willowy woman named Laura, realized I was beginning another miração and she found me a chair and put me at the foot of the cross in the garden. The daime was coming on very strong indeed, and I suddenly felt nauseous with fear and adrift in a dark cloud. Taking out my prayer beads and struggling to seize the tiller of my consciousness, I began my abbreviated form of the rosary.

Ave Maria . . . Ave Maria . . . Ave Maria . . .

Soon my head was tilted back and a warm light was pouring down from above—was I imagining this? Was this really a hand I felt on my forehead?

Margerie, a pilgrim from São Paulo, appeared out of the night, delighted, and pulled up a seat beside me as I was swept into warm colors and light in profound adoration of Santa Maria. Opening my eyes, it was as if they had finally focused: I was in a garden of eternity. The colored lights on the cross that had drawn me upward went out, and a little girl ran up and left a candle burning before us. Through the miração I saw a woman in white kneeling across the way. As Santa Maria began to speak to me, waves of gentleness reached recesses of my heart I had despaired of ever touching. I was crying with joy.

Laura joined us. The women were delighted, stroking my back and laughing with me. Laura sang a hymn to Maria, and then Margerie got excited and, leafing through a book in the darkness, found a hymn of her own. I felt left out because I didn't know a song to Maria.

But then I remembered The Beatles' "Let It Be," and the English lyrics filled the courtyard. It was exquisite, like breathing diamonds and stars out into the universe.

The last time Sean and I saw Luis he took us to his home. Crossing the Rio Branco and walking through the park named after Chico Méndes, we passed the scored rubber trees and entered a small compound of slat-board houses raised up on stilts.

A family was washing themselves at the community water trough as we filed by upon the wooden planks that provided a walkway through the mud. A simple padlock hung at his door, but Luis had forgotten his key. Sean picked it for him, and we entered the tiny space, dominated by a refrigerator, a fan, and an ironing board. A few books sat on his shelf. The room bespoke his voluntary, disciplined frugality. We sat on his bed as Luis poured us glasses of *guarana,* the ubiquitous Brazilian soft drink.

Luis's work was going well. He told us how his plans to set up collectives and train forest workers, allowing them to reap the wealth of the forest while sustaining it for future generations, were meeting acceptance in the new socialist-minded government of President Lula. As well, the power to enforce these new environmental and indigenous rights laws was being granted, without which they would be meaningless.

In my last image of Luis, he is standing with a hymnal in hand, singing for us about the stars guiding us on, about the *caboclos*—helping spirits of the Umbanda spiritual tradition related to the spirit of the natives of the forest—and about Santa Maria, praise arising from the sacred use of *cannibas sativa,* more commonly known as marijuana, to worship the Virgin Mary.

The songs had the simplicity and melodic beauty of medieval plain-chant, as well as its depth of religious feeling. His high, clear voice competed with the television that his neighbors, directly on the other side of the thin slat-board wall that separated their domiciles, had turned on and set blasting. Luis showed no impatience at all.

A buffalo emerged out of the darkness with a slow, stately gait, an apparition of gentle strength in the thick jungle surrounding the Forteleza, a Santo Daime community located in the forest a couple of hours out of Rio Branco. It was two weeks after my visit to the community in Alto Santo, weeks filled with ceremonies that seemed to have anointed my eyes with spirit: the buffalo moved as symbol, both part of and transcendent to the world.

Searching for the Forteleza, we traveled down roads of thick mud, pulling up to *fazendeiros'* shacks to ask directions. The sun had set over the vast, open landscape dotted by cattle and gigantic palm trees as I wondered if we would ever find this elusive "fortress" in the jungle. But we did, and as we ascended a winding path I could see on the horizon above another brilliantly lit open-air structure like the church at Alto Santo. The sound of singing reached our ears, accompanied by the hum of a generator.

Beneath the Caravaca Cross I attempted to scrape the mud off my shoes. The feeling out there was of raw frontier, with only the most basic of essentials. The church floated on its little concrete slab like a postage stamp on a verdant sea. Inside, the scenario was similar to the one at Alto Santo. Men and women danced opposite one another with the maracas, the band jamming away in the center.

But there were differences. Here the men wore business suits—blue slacks and jacket, white shirt, and blue tie. It gave me pause. While the guys in the suits at Alto Santo meant business, the fact the suits were white with a green pinstripe gave them the aspect of a chorus line in a cabaret, taking the edge off of my own Pavlovian reactions to the uniform. These outfits seemed almost evangelical. A little alarm went off in my mind. Suits spell danger: the incarcerating world of the vengeful father.

I was taken to drink. A very ample cup was poured for me. I tossed it down and went and sat, feeling some resistance but not yet clear what it was. I watched the little children of the Forteleza, who danced in their own sections, singing the hymns from memory, and then ran off to play together. Attempting to follow the music, to surrender myself to the experience, I found that the reverse was happening.

The monotony of the singing, the concrete, and the fluorescent lights were all becoming unendurable. *Why can't they use natural lights?* I complained to myself. *It is impossible to travel through fluorescent lights. It's a brick wall into the world of spirit.* Staring at the concrete pad, I felt absolutely cut off from the earth.

Suddenly my body launched me out of the structure, across the lawn, past someone vomiting in the darkness, to the outer perimeter of the compound. Leaning upon a post and looking off into the jungle, I felt torn between worlds. The jungle was out there calling while I was stuck with my obligations within the compound. The human world was pitted against the natural world. As I had done so many times in my life, I leaned against the fence and gazed with yearning into the freedom outside.

My head dropped onto the post. A *miração* washed over me, and I heard the voice of Grandmother Ayahuasca speaking to me. "You have the ability to transform into an animal," she said. "It's a precious gift you have been given, but not everyone can understand it. You can live in both worlds, the human and the animal, and move back and forth without impedance."

Deep in dream, I heard the sound of approaching footsteps behind me. Turning around, I saw two men in suits, *fardadoes*, who had come out for me.

Ah yes, the Brazilian imperative to incorporate into the group. "Yes, I am fine. Quite well, actually. Thank you so much for coming to check on me. I will return momentarily . . . ," I dissembled, but to no avail. I realized they were concerned that in my state a spirit might attack me or I would be led off by a will-o'-the-wisp into the forest. Surrendering, I returned to the safety of the church, but I knew I was radiating foreignness at the moment. I could not sit with the others, and, finding a seat on the outskirts I clutched my prayer beads, holding on for the rest that was to come.

It came hard, waves of repressed material bubbling up and bursting in my mind. It was the *apuração,* the stage of purification, the emptying out of the storehouses of consciousness. Working my prayer beads, struggling toward the light, I found myself gesticulating and grimacing and could imagine what I must have looked like to the watchful fardadoes. But there was nothing for it. I was holding on for dear life.

Then a spirit flashed into my consciousness. A face like Apollo, a superhero in green with an eternal, beautiful, young man's vitality: Hermes, messenger of the gods. His piercing eyes met mine and I knew him, and his hand flashed out and he slapped a jewel into my forehead and was gone.

"A spirit just came and put a jewel in my forehead," I said to myself in the rich silence he had left in his wake. *Cool.*

Jewels, of course, have medicinal properties. As the miração unfolded further, I saw how my masculine life was being subtly warped by my adversarial relationship with my father, how my resisting of his conservative perspectives was preventing the growth of aspects of my own masculinity. I saw the only possible stance toward my father was one of veneration, that I had to allow all superfluous material to fall away. After all, he was the father who had given me life, and through him was one avenue to the Father. Only through acceptance of my own father could I develop as a fully realized male in my own right.

I could stand again, and I went in to join the congregation. As soon as I picked up a maraca to enter the line, the music stopped. As I stood there like the guy who missed the train, someone approached me and took me to meet the *padrinho* (literally, "little father," a term of endearment used for the male elders of the church), Luis Mendez do Nascimento, who had been a disciple of Mestre Irineu's. A small, thin old man with a beaming face, he asked me if the Forteleza had been difficult to find. Pausing, I judiciously answered that it was "well concealed," and we both burst into delighted laughter.

People were taking seats in preparation for something. I found myself seated smack in the middle of the congregation, fully integrated back into the human world, listening to an impassioned, learned disquisition on the economic history of Acre. The speaker, a university professor, orated without notes, focusing his story around the figure of the *seringueiro,* the rubber tapper whose impoverished, solitary existence as well as his heartless exploitation by the capitalists and landowners is remembered and honored at the Forteleza.

It was, I realized, a Marxist analysis—or a Christian one—where the poor worker, the least of men, is the fundament of the entire economic superstructure, and, as the Gospels repeatedly stress, the very person of Christ.

The padrinho sat, his legs crossed like a gentleman, listening with rapt attention, as did the rest of the congregation. As the narrative took up the story of Chico Méndes, delivered with great veneration and a specificity of detail that reflected the depth of grief still existing within the elders of the community, I realized that the man had been speaking for more than two hours and there was still no sign of restlessness in the group. Nor was his energy flagging, unlike my own. The discourse concluded with a vision of humanity's collaboration with the forest, of the salvific power now emerging from it, and of economic justice for all the people of Acre.

Pushing their chairs to the side, the congregation then leaped to their feet and, to reinvigorate themselves, began running laps around the church. Standing to the side watching them race by laughing like children, I was again struck by wonder at this frontier of humanity. Where in the United States, I thought, would people sit and attend to a discourse of such depth and vision about their own community and its future? Had the revolutionaries and visionaries of the thirteen colonies once done the same in their meetinghouses and churches?

The speechifying continued far into the morning. I realized through my exhausted haze that the padrinho was welcoming me to the church. Then to my astonishment, in the ultimate gesture of acceptance of me as a visitor, he cried out, *"Viva os Estados Unidos!"*—"Long Live the United States!" There are few places indeed upon this earth where the common people will still cry out for the long life of the United States of America. But now I understood. It is only through veneration of one another that we can awaken to our own true nature.

The Kaxinawa Indians, the last uncontacted name on the list given to me by the members of the Arca, were sitting in plain view the entire time, but it took me two weeks to notice them. Finally, browsing through the brilliant seed necklaces and bows and arrows in a little trading post in the center of the park in Rio Branco, I took a good look at the Indian behind the counter: small indeed in stature, high cheekbones, jet black hair, a singsong accent to his Portuguese, and a deep sense of self-possession in his brown eyes.

Suddenly inspired, I reached into my backpack and pulled out my journal, flipping hastily to the back pages where I had my list of contacts. "You wouldn't happen to know Fabiano Kaxinawa?" I asked in my clumsy Portuguese.

"Yes. I am him," he responded with amusement.

According to the Kaxinawa, knowledge of ayahuasca was received by their ancestor from a village of anacondas.[3]

A hunter named Yube, seeing an anaconda emerge from a lake and transform into a beautiful woman, made love to her and, returning to her village under the water, married her. There he made a garden, went hunting with his father-in-law, and had three children with his wife. One day his snake wife told him there would be a ceremony with *nixi pai,* ayahuasca, and she warned him not to drink.

"You will become scared and will call out the name of my people and they will kill you." But the hunter drank anyway and then cried out in terror, "The snakes are swallowing me!" In one version, when the hunter cried out his wife coiled herself lovingly around him and began singing sweetly in his right ear. His mother-in-law did the same thing, singing in his left ear. Finally, his father-in-law coiled himself around all three of them and, placing his face upon the hunter's forehead, accompanied the song as well.

Nonetheless, Yube had caused deadly offense to the anacondas and he only managed to escape from the lake with the help of a little bods fish who returned him to his human wife and home.

But the underwater realm eventually reclaimed him: one day walking in a heavy rain his foot slipped into a stream and his anaconda son seized his big toe, followed by his daughter who swallowed his foot, and then his wife who gulped down his whole body up to his armpits, crushing all his bones. Yube remained alive only long enough to instruct the people in the making of the brew and the songs he had learned from the anacondas in the underwater world. He died and, where he was buried, four kinds of ayahuasca grew from his limbs, each of which when drunk in memory of their ancestor show "just a little piece of all there is to know about his and our own life."*

Sean and I returned to Fabiano's trading post to talk with him. This time he was joined by other members of his tribe, all of them young except for a silent older man who just watched. We all sat and I opened our dialogue by asking them, "What is it we can do for you?"

"We open our ceremonies to visitors as part of our desire to share our culture," said Fabiano. "You are welcome to join without obligation." I

---

*An intriguing parallel is offered in ancient Irish folklore. Dian Cecht, the chief physician of the Tuatha De Danaan, the elven people of Irish mythology, slays his son Miach in a frenzy of rage and envy when his son proves more skillful in medicine than he, and he buries him on the plain outside of Tara. By the next day a miraculous growth of herbs had sprung up, outlining Miach's body, every organ and bone and sinew. Each herb had special powers relating to the part of the body from which it had sprung. Airmed, Miach's sister, came to mourn for her brother and she saw the herbs, 365 in all, growing out of his grave. She spread her cloak on the ground and started gathering the herbs to dry them, sorting them out according to their healing properties. But the jealous Dian Cecht came upon her as she was completing the task. He grabbed the cloak and scattered the herbs, mixing them all up together so that it was impossible to sort them out again, and to this day no one person really knows all the healing properties of herbs.[4]

told them I was a writer, and I could help by depicting their lives to the outside world.

They nodded, noncommittal.

Sean asked them about their native village, and they told us it was three days' journey by boat toward the frontier of Peru. Sometimes they take small groups of people there. "Perhaps you will want to go one day," another of the young men said, warming up to Sean and his affinity for the forest.

They gave him a gift of a headband before we departed, woven with an abstract image of a jaguar. "Wear it on your forehead during the ceremony," they told him.

"Man, this is my dream," said Sean as we walked back to the hotel. "To be running around naked in the jungle with a blowgun hunting monkeys with these guys. Can you imagine anything better?"

We gathered later that evening at their kiosk, where we were joined by a small group of other ayahuasca pilgrims: a beautiful Turkish girl I had seen dancing at Alto Santo, a female journalist from northern Brazil who was accompanied by a young man with a guitar, and a guy from São Paulo wearing sandles and white, loose-fitting garments.

The work was held far outside of Rio Branco, at a center the Kaxinawa have created as a bridge between cultures. Recognizing that isolation is no longer an option for them, but also clear that they do not wish to lose themselves in the maelstrom of dislocation and economic anonymity of Brazilian culture, they have opted to become bicultural. The Kaxinawa themselves come to the center to learn Portuguese, how to ride a bicycle, and how to work an ATM and a cellular phone, while non-natives such as ourselves come to be educated in the ways of the Kaxinawa.

Walking through the compound we encountered classrooms with chalkboards and ancestral figures, rough-hewn and primitive to European eyes.

A fear was eating at me as we took our places for the ceremony in an elegant wooden structure with a high-sloped roof of woven palm fronds, a fear that ayahuasca is really just a sort of Prozac, temporarily lifting the mind up but not going to the root of our dilemma. Maybe I was fooling myself and would return to California with some good stories but the same old self. I was weary too of the fundamentalism of Daime, the doctrine, the *salvadores*, the repetition of the word *Jesus*—not as a mantra to enter the divine but as a vaguely oppressive fixture of belief—and the casting of the entire movement into a New Testament mold.

The young guitarist turned out to be a strange bird: a Daime evangelist. His attempts to dominate the group went on until I began grumbling that if I didn't have to hear the word *Jesus* again for a year I wouldn't be at all displeased.

The Kaxinawa sat, patient and vigilant, happily joining in with the songs about our precious savior Jesus. But the Kaxinawa, with their ancient lineage of rainforest medicine, work with ayahuasca (not daime), and I saw that evening that daime is only a brief portion of the vast territory of Grandmother Ayahuasca. The brew they choose is a light one, a very gentle visitation that, when it came, made me put my hands on the earth: on *things*—dear, fresh, particular things—the earth, our ground, to bring me home again.

We wore red stripes on our faces. The young men of the tribe wore headdresses and crowns of feathers, feathers of flight springing from their upper arms. When the evangelical portion of the evening subsided, they sang into the night like an animal sings into it, like the forest sings to itself, in its native tongue, accompanying themselves with flute and maracas. Portuguese and English, even the guitar itself, seemed a rude imposition upon this world, even as we attempted to praise it with our barbaric Indo-European tongues and instruments.

The natives rocked us into the night with invocations and sounds such as we had never encountered before, ending each song with bursts of childlike giggling. At the end of one, Fabiano, who turned out to be an apprentice shaman, explained to us that the entire tribe gathers to sing that particular piece whenever someone is leaving the village for a long journey, to wish them happiness and good fortune on his or her way.

The image of a people gathering to sing for one another, thereby opening and creating a dreaming way through the forest, made me reflect on the cold mechanisms of my own culture, with its straight-cut roads lined with advertisements.

The Turkish girl was wearing a feather headdress and dancing a slow invocation in the center of the room. The seed pods sitting on the table that open in the night for the bats to come and feed were beginning to close. A new day was coming. Sean suddenly appeared at my side, looking worried.

"Man, they want me to play my guitar. What am I gonna do?"

"So, what's the problem?"

"I can't play them 'Mommas Don't Let Your Babies Grow Up to be Cowboys.'"

"Oh yeah, I see your point." I tried to find a way to resolve this dilemma. "Why don't you play them the Villa Lobos Prelude #1?" I said, knowing Sean had been shutting himself up with the work of the Brazilian composer.

"Oh yeah, good idea. I'll give it try."

Sean was not enthusiastic, and played the cello-inspired melody in the bass under strain.

The Kaxinawa politely clapped when he concluded. Maybe they would have liked Willie Nelson better.

In the morning, squinting our eyes against the light now dancing off the lake, we embraced the others and hiked out to await our taxi driver.

Sean was standing in his coat with his hat pulled down over his eyes in a way that reminded me of something.

"You look like a cholo, man!" I laughed.

"Yeah, I thought those guys were really cool when I was a kid. Everybody else hated them but me." Sean, displaying his talent for embodying the mores of other cultures, broke into the stance of the Mexican Americans with their slicked back hair, hair nets and Ben Davis jackets and pants.

We cracked up. "What was that story you once told me about that gang you encountered?" he asked.

"Oh, right. Me and my friend Tyrone were on the street passing the night in that old Greyhound station on Market Street, and these three Mexican guys dressed in black kept cruising through, moving in formation, like sharks." I imitated their sharp, precise movements. "Then just at the moment we cracked up at a joke, they were passing by. All three of them wheeled on us. Perfect, like flamenco dancers. The middle, taller guy leveled his eyes on mine and said, 'What are you laughing at?' I felt nothing but respect for them, so I just raised my hands and said, 'Private joke.' The guy nodded and they turned on a dime and cruised back off again. They had it down."

As we joked a huge white bird cut the early morning sky, a lean aerodynamic ascetic, all stomach and bill, honed to transparency by his habitat. I watched him with awe as he sailed over the forest, from which a rich symphony of sound was now emerging. We and the forest and the albatross all caught up in the same dream of Pachamama.

Many days later, after a grueling riverboat ride up the Rio Madeira to Manaus and a blurred stretch of long hours in the artificial vacuum of air travel, I arrived in San Francisco.

My father, white haired and prosperous looking, was waiting for me. We shook hands and regarded each other through the veil of memories, some of them getting better now. As we wandered through the airport I gave a thumbnail sketch of what I'd been doing.

"Ayahuasca?" he came to a halt. "That's not like peyote, is it?" His voice betrayed his deep suspicion of all things "drugs."

"Yes. In fact, it is," I answered, stopping and looking him squarely in the eye. "I did peyote in the desert in Mexico once. I liked it a lot."

Something in the tone of my voice resolved the issue for my father, and I never heard him react with suspicion to my work with plants again. Instead, he fell silent and gave me the floor.

As we got into the car, he turned down the voice of Rush Limbaugh on the radio. Turning to me, he announced, "Boy, I'm gonna play you the finest music ever recorded," and held up a CD with a flourish. It went into the machine and out came the walking bass of Elvis's "Heartbreak Hotel."

I was pleasantly startled. I had no memories of my father ever playing music for sheer enjoyment, much less expressing enthusiasm for rock 'n' roll. *We're talkin' the same language here,* I thought.

As we settled onto the freeway he started to reminisce about his childhood.

"I remember when Elvis first came on television. It was the Tommy and Jimmy Dorsey Show, but nobody saw it and the next day at school you would have thought nothing had happened."

"Why?" I asked, intrigued at this glimpse I was getting into my father's background.

"It was a big band jazz show, and none of the kids watched it. But a week later he went on Ed Sullivan and did that thing with his hips and suddenly the whole world was talking about it."

Shit, I thought, *my father lived through that junction in music history and marked it.* "What else do you remember, Dad?" I prompted him.

"I had a friend, Eric Stanton, who lived right around the corner from me. He was a good guy, married, had a couple of kids. You know, the whole Ward and June Cleaver thing. Anyway, his wife, Jean, went crazy when she heard Elvis. She played his music all day long, put pictures of him in every room, and then one day she just up and vanished. Left a note saying she was going to go follow Elvis. Left her kids and everything. Eric never heard from her again."

"That's wild," I commented. There was a relish in my father's story-telling, about the events of his surburban life, that I didn't know he had. "So what happened to poor Eric?"

"He raised the kids on his own. I lost track of him after a few years, but I assume he got remarried."

We listened to one of Elvis's gospel numbers. "Elvis was a very simple, deeply spiritual man," my father sighed.

This is great, I sat there thinking. *This just beats all. . . .*

4 CLOSE TO THE HURT LIES GROWING THE BALM

If you bring forth what is within you,
what is within you will save you. If you
do not bring forth what is within you,
what you do not bring forth will destroy
you.

THE GOSPEL OF THOMAS, SAYING 70

Upon a hilltop, above the lights of Rio de Janeiro, is a little church called Jardim Praia da Beira Mar where, nestled amid massive boulders of granite, is a platform upon whose floor is drawn a star. Within that pentagram, dressed in white, celebrants dance, facing into the center where there rests an altar with images of the Virgin Mary, Jesus, and the founders of the Santo Daime.

On my long, winding journey home from the Amazonian state of Acre, I visited the church to join the dance a final time before catching my plane back to the United States. I was welcomed there, along with a small group of visiting Cariocas, by its director, Nilton Caparelli.

Caparelli, as he is familiarly called, is a white-haired gentleman who wears wire-rimmed glasses and a benevolent expression upon features suggesting some steel in the backbone. This quality I later watched emerge as he orchestrated the arrival of spirits at the *mesa branca,* or white table ceremony, he conducted that evening.

Caparelli told us a story, a parable that perfectly encapsulated a thing I had struggled to clarify while journeying among the Daime communities in Acre: addiction and its relation to medicine.

This is the story I heard, or as my imagination embellished it.

In the final days of the Incan empire, as the Spaniards' guns, germs, and steel laid waste to the world below, a last vestige of The People surrounding the Royal Inca withdrew to a mountain fastness, vanishing from the sight of the foreign conquistadors. There, in a high city of stone, the Incans began their migration to the next world, from where they would await their appointed time to return to this world again.

Overseeing this transmigration was a priest named Ayahuasca, who also took care that his knowledge of the medicine was communicated to the many tribes of the Amazon before their departure.

As the Incans dreamt of the sacred city of gold, word leaked out to the conquistadors scouring the country below. This rumor of a golden city, surpassing in wealth even the navel of the world, Cuzco, whose temples they had stripped and whose people they had tortured and enslaved, awakened further ambition for conquest. El Dorado, they named it, and assembling armies they marched out into the jungle to find it.

Dying of malaria, their armor rusting and their horses devoured, they sought the sacred realm with the edge of their sword and it eluded them, leaving them stranded, starved, mad, wandering lost in the worlds below, and finally dead.

Those few who did come, after many years of searching, upon the high city of stone found only mummies and clay vessels, the cast-off husks of the Incans' successful transmigration. In their bitterness, they destroyed them, without comprehending that the traces of the City of Gold lay at their feet.

As Caparelli unfolded his tale, compassion for the Spaniards stirred within me.

Taken as history, I questioned the account's veracity, but as a teaching story it struck deep. In the Incans, I saw the path of renunciation available through disciplined, ceremonial work with teacher plants. In the Spaniards and their attempts to violently seize gold, I saw the path of addiction. (In fact, the native peoples of America, who never valued gold beyond its ceremonial worth, wondered if the Spaniards secretly ate it.)

Is not the plunging of the needle into the vein, at root, nothing but a desperate expression of the desire for self-transcendence? Wandering like the ghost of a conquistador in lower realms, the addict attempts to seize the "high" contained in a white powder. But that heavenly ascent is a counterfeit of the golden bliss of liberation that comes with renouncing the addiction to the self and all its meticulous, finely woven, and subtle delusions.

This was more than an intellectual concern of mine—my brother had died homeless, struggling with the dark entities in substances. My sister bottomed out in a prison cell, and then arose after completing the twelve-step program of Narcotics Anonymous to become a formidable drug counselor and advocate for the rights of substance abusers. And until entheogens intervened in my career, I too had been bound for an early grave in the clutch of substances—such had been my appetite for self-transcendence.

Was it possible, I asked myself, that medicinal plants, especially entheogens, could be systematically effective in treating addiction? Could our abuse of plants—tobacco, alcohol, sugar, cocaine, crack, heroin, marijuana—be counteracted by the therapeutic intervention of the innate intelligence in plants?

Had not my vision of the vine told me, "Close to the hurt lies growing the balm"?

I confess that, at first, I did little to follow up on my pet theory. I learned that native peoples have long been quietly employing plant medicines to successfully heal alcoholism among their own people, but it has attracted sparse attention from the medical establishment. For example, the ritual use of the mescaline cactus San Pedro on the Peruvian coast has met with a high rate of success (around 60 percent after five years), and peyote and tobacco have been used to significantly reduce alcoholism among Native Americans in the United States and Canada.[1] Ibogaine, a plant native to Africa and utilized in the Bwiti religion, has also demonstrated remarkable effectiveness in treating heroin, alcohol, and cocaine addiction.

But the analytical approaches of scientific researchers and their attempts to patent the curative powers of plants turned me off.*

As well, I found the proponents of psychedelic therapies for addiction, with their promises of "inner transformative journeys," distasteful. Missing was the ecological consciousness, the sense of community and the humility and gratitude toward nature, that I had encountered among the churches of Brazil. Without integration into a native cosmology, I was suspicious that the outcome would be just another drug experience, lacking the reframing of individuality from the perspective of the sacred.

---

*For example, Howard Lotsof, searching for a psychedelic experience in 1962, took ibogaine, but he found instead he'd kicked his heroin addiction without suffering from the classic symptoms of withdrawal. He went on to patent the molecule and a method of treatment, claiming he had "discovered" the plant's medicinal properties. As he states it, "The keys to marketing any pharmaceutical product are patent protection, proper financing and a clear understanding of the regulatory requirements which must be met. The Endabuse Procedure™ in which ibogaine may be used to interrupt heroin, cocaine, alcohol, or nicotine addiction are the only research areas for which NDA International will supply ibogaine for human treatment."[2] While his attempts to control access are understandable in light of the hysteria unleashed by recreational use of LSD—another pharmaceutical product that proved to be remarkably effective in therapeutic contexts—his approach to the plant removes it from its sacred context and the ancestral wisdom embedded in traditional practices. Consequently, ibogaine runs the risk of becoming just another denatured drug for sale.

So I left these thoughts to simmer on the back burner, thinking my pilgrimage was complete. Then the course of my work—and life—changed in encountering Susana.

The defining moment came at La Peña in Berkeley, an artistic center founded by Chileans in exile from the Pinochet regime, at an art opening where images of ayahuasca played a significant role. Wandering among the pictures, I found the vine interwoven in the artist's mythos with scenes of liberation for indigeous people. But then I noticed the world was sharply divided between the browns and the whites, and the whites, I realized with a chill, all wore uniforms with swastikas.

My host pointed out Susana, a young Chilean woman who sat before a microphone tuning her guitar, telling me she was a clinical psychologist who had worked for many years in programs for the prevention of drug addiction in Chile. She had come to the States to do Ph.D. research on the healing effects of ayahuasca. Her interest particularly lay in the *icaros,* the songs used to direct the helping spirits of *curanderos,* or shamans, in their work upon the patient.

Looking at her, her graceful movements and petite form were suddenly engraved on my mind, and when we were introduced I saw her high cheekbones and the way her eyes seemed to take in everything with a warm, active intelligence and I thought, *This is the kind of woman I love.*

But I was uncertain of my welcome. Susana was ensconced in a different world. While I understood Chilean anger against northern militaries (their democratic government having been overthrown by a Nixon administration sponsored coup d'etat), I was uncomfortable about having the only representatives of my genetic background depicted as Nazi on the walls around me. We spoke briefly and then she excused herself for the sound check. I departed.

The next time I saw her, we were part of a circle that gathered in a lodge in the coastal redwoods to work with a shaman teaching in the Andean tradition of Peru. Susana didn't remember me, but I did her.

In the circle I never quite managed to get her attention. Her demeanor had "professional" written all over it, managerial. But I also noticed the care with which she would light a candle to the Virgin at just the right moment, how quick she was to dance and sing. And when she shared with the group, her words were more than finely crafted: they were playful and embracing. I found myself wanting to know that beautiful thing in the depths of her. The one exchange we had before she finally noticed me was in the kitchen right after a session.

"It was very subtle tonight," I told her, reflecting. "No powerful visions, just teaching about how to be in my body."

"Good!" she said, and walked briskly away.

Then the moment of recognition came. Having just returned from my pilgrimage through the ayahuasca churches in Brazil, I drove up through the forest to attend a weekend at the lodge. Parking my old pickup truck, I put on my battered Australian wide-brimmed hat and walked through the rain to the house. As usual, I was late.

The front door swung open. There stood Susana. She looked at me as if she were seeing something she hadn't before.

"You look like . . ."

I saw it. Brown hat, leather jacket, necklace with the symbol of the monkey carved by the Kaxinawa Indians . . .

". . . Indiana Jones!" she concluded.

We laughed merrily. She had finally noticed me. The words of the medium channeling the preta velha in the Barquinha church in Brazil flashed through my mind. I suddenly suspected the partner I had been searching for was standing before me.

Susana first discovered the healing power of the voice during the Pinochet dictatorship in Santiago, Chile, which lasted from 1974 to 1990. "What you have during a dictatorship is silence. You cannot talk. Singing songs was the way to express and to denounce the injustices of the time. Singing in *peñas,* in public sites, the collective pain and hope for change, gave me a sense of purpose and a means to do something," she told me.

She was also risking her life. The dictatorship took the threat of music seriously. In the first roundups after the capitulation and death of deposed president Salvadore Allende, they cut off the hands of the great folksinger Victor Jara in the Santiago stadium.

Susana went on to train in music therapy to bring that healing power into her work as a clinical psychologist. But what awoke her interest in the icaros—the songs of the shamans that come as gifts from the spirits of the plants—was her own personal experience of healing years before at Takiwasi, a center for the treatment of addiction that utilizes indigenous healing practices.

The origins of Takiwasi, located in Tarapoto, Peru, lie in 1986 when Dr. Jacques Mabit, a Frenchman, and his Peruvian wife, Dr. Rosa Giove, began their investigations, through observation and participation in the work of Amazonian curanderos, into the ritual use of medicinal plants in the treatment of consumers of crack cocaine, marijuana, cocaine, and alcohol. They came to conclude that indigenous medicine, whose origins some anthropologists claim lie depicted in the Magdalenian cave art of seventeen thousand years ago, offers a powerful methodology to open realms of healing unutilized by Western medicine.*

In 1992 Takiwasi opened its doors to offer a protocol of attention to consumers of legal and illegal drugs. The protocol combines Western psychology and medicine with indigenous *curanderismo*.†

Susana first went to the center seeking a cure for symptoms that arose after her initiatory session of ayahuasca in Chile. Led by an inexperienced guide, her journey had spun out of control into a relentless twelve-hour Mr. Toad's Wild Ride through the infinite dimensions of the cosmos.

---

*Actually, we now know the practice of medicine predates our species: "At Shanidar Cave in Iraq, the skeleton of a Neanderthal was found buried with seven medicinal species of plants placed in a ring around the body."[3]

†Curanderismo is a healing tradition widespread throughout Latin America, but the mestizo curanderismo, or vegetalismo, practiced at Takiwasi "is a Peruvian shamanistic tradition that evolved from indigenous Amazon practices and cosmologies progressively permeated by Western elements, due to factors involved in the acculturation and disintegration of native groups. Vegetalistas address the physical, psychosomatic, and psychosocial healing requests of a vast urban poor and rural population that still harbors strong indigenous elements."[4]

Afterward, she began having very strange symptoms: shaking, sweating, dizziness, fever, disorientation, and sudden expansions and contractions of consciousness. She awoke at night shaking like a leaf, a feeling of energy rampaging in her body seeking release. Finally, it was identified as rising kundalini, the energy of consciousness so familiar to Eastern traditions of yogic practice. She had a blockage at her heart chakra.

The first person she met on the pleasant grounds of Takiwasi was a small, thin old shaman named Don Solon whose face radiated kindness. He said to her, "Oh, you got left nervous. It's certain a serpent got left inside your body," and he invited her to be healed by him. So she went in the early morning to his little house inside of Takiwasi where he sang, beat a *shacapa*—a fan of medicinal leaves—over her, and blew tobacco and perfume on her. Of that experience Susana says, "I felt a lot of love for this old guy, and everyone also told me about the power of his icaros and how much love he put into the sessions through his voice."

Her symptoms began to improve, but she needed to be guided back into the realm of ayahuasca to emerge with a complete cure. "In the session I was very scared. It was only my second and the first one in Chile had been so deep and difficult. When the ayahuasca started coming inside I started to sweat and felt superhot, but also really content with the songs, the circle, the sounds of the jungle containing the experience. It was perfect."

Then she started to journey into the realm of the plants, as if they were all part of a single, great tree, discovering their different levels, entering them and visiting the beings inside them. She had many encounters in the various branches, but there was a feeling of not going any further, and she felt disoriented and tense. Finally the individual healings began, and she heard Rosa Giove calling her name to come to the center of the circle. "I went forward and she started to sing the 'Icaro de la A,'" she said.

By the time Susana related this history to me at Takiwasi, I had heard that icaro, and it had struck me like a love song to the heart, its serpentine melody filled with yearning and summoning:

Ábrete corazón, ábrete sentimiento	Open heart! Open emotion!
Ábrete entendimiento	Open understanding!
Deja a un lado la razón	Leave to one side reason
Y deja brillar el sol	And allow the sun to shine
Escondido en tu interior.	Hidden in your interior.
Ábrete memoria antigua	Open ancient memory!
Escondida en la tierra, en las plantas,	Hidden in the earth,
En el viento, bajo el agua	In the plants and wind,
	Beneath the waters.
Es tiempo ya	It's time now
Ya es ahora	This is the moment
Ábrete corazón y recuerda	Open heart! And remember
Como el espíritu cura	How spirit cures,
Como el amor sana	How love heals
Como el árbol florece	How the tree flourishes
Y la vida perdura.	And life endures.
Abre tus alas	Open your wings
Respira profundo	breathe deeply
Y elévate hasta el cielo	And rise to the sky
Como las águilas	Like the eagles
No tengas temor	Have no fear
Confía en ti, confía en Dios	Trust in yourself, trust in God
Confía en la vida	Trust in life.

"The moment she started singing '*ábrete corazón*,'" Susana continued, "I felt she knew exactly what was going on with my blockage in the heart area and she was singing into it with such love. And it was a woman singing. It was so compassionate and intimate I felt like anything I was holding in my heart just melted with her song and I remember just crying and crying and a great release of tension. Then I went back to my place and I started having a deep journey into the tree of life, a huge tree, and I was in the center of the tree, inside, in a place that was very warm, protected, like a womb, and I entered a cycle of my getting pregnant, and when the baby was born it came out and was absorbed by the tree and went out to the branches and then something came back to the tree through the roots and I got pregnant again, and the cycle continued thousands of times, producing life, life was flowing, letting the energy flow from the base to the top. It was the release of the blockage of the kundalini.

"I got two things out of the experience," she told me, adopting her researcher's mode. "The first is the importance of the proper setting, a ritual space oriented toward the sacred, and preferably in a community that holds similar healing intentions. The second is the importance of the bond with an experienced guide. This is someone who understands proper dose, can provide a safe, structured container that feels familiar to the client, and whose mediation anchors their experience and helps them integrate it. The core of this relationship is expressed through the voice mediating the power of ayahuasca, through a song where the shaman says to you, 'I know what is going on. I am with you. I want the best for you.' The shaman says to the ayahuasca, 'Mother, come help this sister. Be good to her.' That it is finally the soul connection in ayahuasca, between two human beings, that heals."

She learned in that session and subsequent ones that the songs of the curanderos work inside the body, calming, directing, and mediating between the extremely powerful effects of the plant and those seeking healing, helping to translate that power into something possible to digest, control, and navigate through.

Her professional interest aroused, she sought through the literature for studies on the experience of healing by participants in ceremonies of ayahuasca, especially related to the function of icaros. She found the healing function of icaros addressed in anthropological literature mainly from the perspective of the shamans, or *vegetalistas,* but not systematically and in depth from the experience of the clients.

Takiwasi offered the perfect environment to realize such a study, with its resident population, developed infrastructure, and therapeutic program already in place—and Jacques Mabit proved welcoming to her project. Susana designed her Ph.D. research, and was nearing her point of departure when I returned from Brazil, having met the jaguar. She liked what she saw.

I did too. Arriving at the confluence of my love of plants with my awakening love of Susana, I chose to follow the river. At the end of the semester, I prepared to resign my teaching position and say farewell to friends and my little cabin in the woods in order to accompany Susana to Takiwasi.

But first, worried that I was losing perspective, I consulted with my father. I expected to hear a conservative argument against rushing off into the Amazon jungle. Instead, his moustache bristling, he said to me, "If you don't take this opportunity, you'll regret it for the rest of your life."

That clinched it. I bought my ticket and completed my preparations to return to the indigenous world of South America.

Takiwasi (the "House of Song" in Quechua) lies in the province of San Martín in Peru, just outside the sleepy but watchful town of Tarapoto. The emerald green mountains surrounding the town, hosting rainbows and lazily circled by vultures, are the site of intense cultivation of the coca plant, which, until recently, made the province one of the primary zones in the world for the production and consumption of cocaine and its derivatives. At the same time, this region of the upper Amazon still possesses great biodiversity, forming the basis for the native medical practices researched by Takiwasi as highly effective therapies in the treatment of addiction.

As I walked down Takiwasi's sandy paths beneath huge spreading trees, through medicinal gardens with carefully labeled plants, my first impression of it was that of a plantation. A soccer field, a carpentry shop, big circular structures with thatched roofs, laboratories, and offices lay spread out on the ample grounds. Just behind the property flowed the river Shilcayo, where a little chapel in the form of a dodecahedron, crowned by a steep thatched conical roof with a totem pole at its summit, rested on stilts. A bell by the entrance called employees and patients to Mass. Inside, the patron of Takiwasi, the Virgin de la Puerta, sat enthroned.

Noticeably absent were any touches of a spiritual New Age community. There were no wind chimes, no crystals rotating in the sunshine.

The founder of Takiwasi, Jacques Mabit, is a cultural phenomenon with strong allies and much opposition. At our first meeting, I encountered a man with Gallic features and gray sideburns, probably in his early fifties, who brought the air of the Sorbonne into the jungle. Having been informed by Susana that he spoke English, I introduced myself in that language and delivered greetings to him from the head of a community in Brazil. To my dismay, he did not respond, but stood boring into me with his intense blue eyes instead.

Hastily backtracking, I apologized in Spanish and reintroduced myself. Warming up, he welcomed me to the center (I abandoned English for the rest of my stay). Mabit turned out to be a gracious host during our stay there.

In the research I had done before leaving for Takiwasi, I learned that Mabit is one of the few practitioners of Western science to train themselves in indigenous medicine. Such a combination of methodologies threatens to behave like a shotgun marriage. For centuries, scientists and priests have ridiculed indigenous ways of knowing with their direct apprehension of disease as primarily spiritual in origin. Yet Mabit champions the rigorous empiricism of the traditional healers, putting it on par with the methods of Western science.

According to Mabit, the visionary effects of ayahuasca, presently stigmatized as hallucinogenic, actually "symbolically manifest the contents of the unconscious." Far from being wanderings of the mind, the visionary effects permit "the rapid extraction of extremely rich and highly coherent psychological material, which can then be worked through various psychotherapeutic methods."

In his scientific framework, "the effects of ayahuasca are not merely visual, but embrace the entire perceptual spectrum, as well as the non-rational functions tied to the right brain and to the paleoencephal or so-called reptilian brain." Coming as it does from the patient's entire spectrum of consciousness, "the patient's clinical experience fosters the development of not only the projective but also the integrative functions of symbolization, authorizing the progressive readjustment of personality structures."

In other words, in crossing the threshold into the realm of the plant, "users are guided into liminal, or symbolically transitional, experiences in which they visit their interior gods and demons . . . which touch depths that could be transcultural by virtue of reaching universal psychological complexes (love, hate, rejection, abandon, fear, peace, etc.)." According to Mabit, the accompanying psychotherapy at Takiwasi allows the patient to understand and integrate the sessions, and then move forward, with fresh questions, in their lives.[5]

Integral to this approach is holding addiction as a thwarted spiritual quest, an interpretation that for me, as an ex-addict, lay especially close to my heart. In this radical interpretation, the disease is best cured at its root: the addict's suffering of the meaningless of his existence. His error lies not in his goal to transcend himself, but in his approach, which inevitably submerges him in ever-deepening cycles of suffering. By providing a sacred container, Takiwasi claims to allow the addict to embark anew on his quest to discover the core truths of his particular existence.

Statistically, the approach has proved to be effective. Takiwasi reports a success rate of 67 percent among those clients who have completed its basic nine-month treatment program.*

Recovery rates vary widely in standard addiction rehabilitation programs—and numbers are often subject to fudging—but an abysmally low 15 percent recovery rate is generally the norm. It is worth emphasizing that the most successful programs, such as Alcoholics Anonymous or Narcotics Anonymous, have a strong spiritual component.

---

*These figures are based on a study of the first seven years of activity at Takiwasi, of patients who completed at least one month of treatment and with at least two years of time out of the clinic—a sample of 211 courses of treatment.[6] It should be added that all patients leave free of any postresidential medication.

I had also heard tales of the treatment at Takiwasi going awry, of patients abandoned in amplified and disturbed states of mind to sort things out on their own. For the moment, however, I was putting such rumors to the side.

My intention was not to go into "treatment." As a writer, my investigations into the healing potentials of ayahuasca had been in the light-filled, celebratory spaces of the Brazilian churches of Daime. I imagined an analogous experience was in store for me.

After all, a passage of twenty years separated me from my struggle with drugs. It came as a terrible surprise, therefore, to learn I had merely buried my past, not resolved it.

Life is simple at Takiwasi, as it is in all of rural Peru, and to be admitted as a patient would be, for a Westerner accustomed to certain standards of comfort, analogous to entering boot camp or a monastery. Patients live communally in a type of barracks, reflecting the general level of poverty of the country. Most of the patients in residence are men, and many are young, and although the goal of Takiwasi is to adapt to persons of different cultural contexts, a monolingual speaker of English would have to learn Spanish rapidly to benefit from the experience.

Near Takiwasi Susana and I rented a small house with a reputation for being *cargada*—charged—from the succession of shamans who had lived there. What attracted us was the garden, a little chunk of jungle filled with plants with *madres*, "power plants": ayahuasca vines; datura trees with their pendant, fluted-bell-shaped flowers; yawar panga vines; coca bushes; and a massive ojé tree spreading its tentacle-like roots like a great octopus through the shallows of the sandy Amazonian soil. A San Pedro cactus, sacred to the shamans of the Andes, sat in a pot by the doorway. The priest who came to bless the house sprinkled holy water upon it, saying, "Oh, this is a very good plant."

Like all sleepy Latin American towns, the surface of the earth was a barnyard. Dogs and chickens wandered through and a pair of incongruous white rabbits hopped about and lay curled up together in the shade.

But the air still belonged to the Amazon, and brilliantly colored birds, foreign to my eyes because of their unique adaptations to the jungle, flitted through. Flowers of strange and marvelous aspect bloomed just down the road. Giant palms supported by buttresses swayed. The Shilcayo flowed nearby, running high from the heavy rains that fell in that season. Emerald green venomous snakes slithered across the dirt roads.

Between the barking of dogs, the crowing of roosters, and the salvos of pulsing Cumbia music playing on cheap stereo systems, a universe of strange sound and communication surrounded us, buzzing and humming and chirping.

Susana was in her element at Takiwasi, and starting putting in long hours doing therapy and conducting holotropic breathwork sessions with the residents, leaving me idling in the garden. I couldn't blame her. As a therapist, the possibility of exploring the patient's integration process of their insights after a ceremony with ayahuasca was unique. But for myself as a writer, I found myself whiling away my time in the garden and wondering what had happened to our romance.

Fortunately, due to its remote locale, Takiwasi is always on the lookout for talent, and I soon found myself integrated into the therapeutic work of the center as a volunteer instructor of Buddhist meditation. In my first encounter with the patients I told them a story from my own history as an addict, something I hoped would help bridge the gap between our different cultures. There were around a dozen of them, with features ranging from indigenous to Nordic. Most were Peruvian, and some showed the marks of having been incarcerated. On the other hand, some of the French patients had the refinement of young men attending salons.

Addiction has many faces. This one was one of mine: In the absence of the sacred, the soul creates its shadow rituals. . . . Our sanctuary was an empty lot, somewhere off Mission Street, nearby an Arab liquor store that would look the other way and sell minors cheap gin. A passed-over place, a space defined by adjacent buildings offering no shelter: pure enclosure, anonymous and purposeless. Broken glass coated the pavement. A set of concrete stairs led to a permanently locked metal door, a light allegorical touch as well as a place to sit. Mean faces somewhere behind every wall, but not a window to gaze down upon our poor theatre.

There the bottle of gin would be broached and passed from hand to hand, or would simply stay before me if I had come for a solitary retreat.

Strange visions, eruptions of violence, uncontrollable laughter, surges of sexual energies, tearful confessions wrenched from the depths, and above all a sense of belonging would follow. Of having dissolved the boundaries to communion, of soaring into the sun of self-immolation.

Then I would wake where I had fallen, remembering dimly, or not at all, how I had ended up in a jail cell or lying in the bushes alongside the sidewalk, a stream of pedestrians flowing by behind me. I always felt cold after the alcohol had ebbed away. And I always returned to that empty lot to uncap the energies within that bottle.

Submerging myself deeper, my hands trembling as I raised the first shot of the morning to my lips, even my friends of the needle and bottle expressed concern. I laughed. The bottle was my self-transcendence— what did the breaking down of my body matter?

And then one day, hanging out near the amphitheater at Tamalpias High School in Mill Valley, word reached me Tyrone wanted to speak with me.

Tyrone was one of the kids who lived in our group home. Curious, I climbed the back steps of the school to find him standing carefully outside the school bounds, holding a large brown paper bag in his arms. With a conspirator's grin, he reached into the bag and began scooping handfuls of dried brown mushrooms with golden caps into another bag.

"Deal!" he said.

Walking to the nearest payphone, I called my group home in Corte Madera and announced this school thing wasn't working and I was heading out. And head out I did, with only my clothes on my back and a giant bag of Psilocybe cubensis *mushrooms stuffed in my backpack.*

Making my pilgrimage from party to party and "experience" to "experience," I became aware that the plant, besides creating incredible, magical effects in my consciousness, was teaching me. For the first time in my life I was apprenticing to something, communing with an intelligence ranked somewhere among the hierarchy of the sacred. It was strangely familiar. Like a birthright.

And then the healing came. It arrived as I stood in my usual pose, bottle in hand, leaning in a doorframe, gazing into a room covered with the bodies of tripping punk rockers. The colors of the guitar of Jimi Hendrix crested and broke in our minds as wavelets touched shore from an ocean of eternity. Ambrosial. Blissful with the million true sounds of the universe. The gods danced. Endless. Free of suffering.

Then I saw it.

"Look at me!" I suddenly announced to the room. "This is me! The guy with the bottle in his hand, leaning in the door, looking in!" The room regarded me momentarily and then withdrew back into its dream again.

I saw the persona I was wearing with perfect clarity, the one that was going to drink himself into the gutter and die there. In the light of eternity unleashed by the mushrooms, I was just a dream among dreams, a brief dance as insubstantial as a cloud drifting through the sky—a blissfully empty sky.

There was nothing to do but to be what I was. There was no other task in this world. All ways led to the embrace of God.

The vision faded as first the coldness of the streets and then the police closed in on me. Gravity finally dashed me to the hard earth, and once again the routine of incarceration—that dull stupidity of fluorescent lights, somnolent televisions, linoleum floors and Formica tabletops—dominated my life.

But I was different somehow, and I finally realized how. Without having the least impulse to reform or "get on the wagon," I had ceased to drink. Tallying up the dates, I concluded with wonder that I hadn't been seriously drunk for a month.

Without seeking it, I had stumbled into a healing experience. Having finally tasted an authentic belonging within spirit, my desperation for the oblivion of the bottle was quenched. At that moment, the cell doors and barred Plexiglas windows vanished, and it felt as if the wing of a passing eagle brushed my face.

When I concluded the men sat in a polite silence in the circle. Finally, a young Frenchman, who had been weighing me with his haunted angelic eyes, spoke up: "You were very lucky, you know. None of us received such gifts. We've had to take the harder road."

One who had taken the harder road was Raphael.

Raphael was in "isolation," which at Takiwasi meant living alone, in a little cottage on the grounds, in order to have a chance to catch up on one's self-reflection. But it was a rigorous self-reflection.

A user since the age of eleven, he was now a young man in his early twenties, with a natural enthusiasm, and a fervent desire to connect. He seemed to be smiling all the time, like an employee in a five-star hotel, and to be interested in everything. It was hard for me to comprehend Susana's description of the desperation that underlay his suave exterior—that his gentility was a mask covering terror, and he struggled with suicidal thoughts and deep depression.

To my eyes, he seemed full of potential and life. It was a hard dilemma, because it wasn't a lack of moral "fiber" that had turned Raphael to cocaine, nor was he a creep wearing a little spoon on a gold chain around his neck. Cocaine was his life rope.

"Cocaine makes you feel you can do everything, you're a huge guy, you've got power. If you're in deep depression, it takes you into a high where everything is fabulous," Susana told me.

"So what's the difference between cocaine and Prozac, anyway?" I asked, suddenly irritated at our hypocrisy in dosing millions with antidepressants while scapegoating others who were engaged in essentially the same activity, only illegally.

"Well, one obvious difference is the level. Prozac doesn't give you the same high cocaine does and doesn't alter consciousness as much. With cocaine you can feel God," she said without blinking.

The problem was, Raphael had a narcissistic wound that thwarted all his efforts to contain his anxiety and terror, a black hole within himself he inevitably orbited back in to. And he had not yet developed the ego structure to support the awful work of dwelling in the dark unknowing until healing occurred. As was common for some addicts, his sessions with ayahuasca had been black for months. No visions, no relief. He had purged, had dieted in the jungle, had done the psychotherapy, but still he didn't seem to be emerging from the black hole.

Finally in desperation he made contact with a local *ayahuasquero,* a magician, and stole out of Takiwasi in the night to drink the brew with him.

The heavens had opened under the magician's guidance, filling him with ecstasy, sending him soaring free from the gravitational pull of the black hole. Returning the following morning to Takiwasi, he was walking on air, but the effect was only temporary, as all magic is.

He crashed into the gravest depression, the dark hole pulling him back in with a vengeance.

The incident illustrated the difficulty of the work done at Takiwasi, where patients are not suppressed with drugs and television, nor brainwashed with ideologies and kept in lockdown. Takiwasi relies instead on the inherent tendency of the psyche to move toward wholeness, a growth process that, like the sprouting of a seed, cannot be rushed. The seed needed more nourishment in Rafael. In his extreme state, without the certainty of a deep stirring of growth, he had bolted for a quick fix.

The therapeutic team rallied. It was Raphael's third treatment at Takiwasi, and it was time to intervene decisively. A two-week program of ergotherapy (such as baking bread and gardening for the community), psychotherapy, and focused self-reflection was designed for him and I was put in charge of teaching him meditation an hour every day.

Essentially, the team was rushing in to build him a self, to put in the foundation stone his ego lacked. This absence of a foundation stone, from the perspective of psychoanalytic theory, is called a "narcissistic wound" and lies at one of the earliest strata of the individual's psychological development. This stage, when the movement away from primary narcissism— where *all things* are the baby's self—to the more individuated awareness of self *and other* occurs, always involves pain. But, if the conditions for the separation are not favorable, say, the baby is left dwelling in unsatisfied, basic needs for a long time, the harshness of deprivation, the thanatos energy related to death, becomes primary in the self. (See the suggestive account later in this chapter, of Francisco's vision of a dark spirit entering his chest as he lay in the cradle.) The problem that arises under extreme conditions in this stage of separation is the energies of eros and thanatos don't become healthily balanced.

According to Melanie Klein there are two possible stances a baby can then adopt toward life.[7] First, there is the depressive stance, where we recognize we have lost something and mourn it passively, under which conditions the personality structure can evolve as more solid and mature. The second is the schizo-paranoid, where the outside becomes monstrous, and as adults we experience deep terrors and a feeling of being devoured by a threatening environment that we cannot completely differentiate from ourselves, pushing us into extreme conditions of autistic withdrawal or overwhelming persecutory fantasy.

The schizo-paranoid stance is a very primary structure, probably the one Raphael was struggling with, and it often underlies heavy addiction. Cocaine gives power back to the subject. Heroin tends to fuse subject and object, returning the addict to an early stage of development before the differentiation between subject and object.

Doped up or not, it's a Sisyphean row to hoe.

Approaching Raphael's cabin for our morning session, I saw he was already out setting up our meditation cushions. He looked up and waved, happy to receive some company.

This was our morning ritual. Each day we sat together in silence, rigorously maintaining the meditation posture, working with the impulsivity of the human body and mind. Raphael, like many addicts, had a strong thirst for spirituality. As a child he discovered the Hari Krishnas down the street and converted his entire family to vegetarianism, and his father to the practice itself.

There was something thrilling in watching his process, how with the yoke of discipline finally settled on his neck, Raphael was a racehorse given full rein in an open field. He luxuriated in focused work on his spirit.

One day he stood up and promptly fell over on his face. Maintaining the seated meditation posture against all obstacles, his legs had fallen asleep without his realizing it. Another day he appeared with a copy of a classic Zen Buddhist text, the Ox-Herding Pictures, he had found in the library and asked me for a full explanation of the medieval Chinese text.

As the sessions flowed by, a sort of feedback loop formed between us. I sat with the Raphael within me, the young addict struggling to tame his impulses and wildly veering thoughts. And as I modeled the disciplined entry into spirit, I became the calming presence of a spiritual father for Raphael, the one he had attempted to invoke in converting his biological one. Then, watching him absorbing the father's stabilizing wisdom, I felt it ripening in me too.

I rang the bell to end the meditation session. Raphael disentangled his legs and then studied me.

"Susana told me you're purging with yawar panga this afternoon."

I nodded my head.

His eyes lit up from within. "I've purged with that plant six times. It's strong. You're getting your initiation today, my friend." He clapped me on the shoulder. "Now you're going to be one of us."

As I lay in the garden in my hammock a few days earlier, a beaming Susana had appeared and announced she had scheduled us for a rigorous series of purges with plants such as yawar panga, azucena, and Rosa Sisa. I gave her a blank look.

I thought purging was for ancient Romans in their vomitoriums.

Of course, my work in the Brazilian churches of Daime had taught me that purging is an important aspect of work with an entheogenic plant, but they had never actually suggested undergoing a purge for its own sake. But having already sat at the lunch table at Takiwasi and listened to conversations of all kinds of bodily fluids and toxins being weirdly mixed with spiritual and psychological concepts, I shouldn't have been surprised.

As Susana had put it to me, "In the mestizo cosmology, there is no separation between body and soul: the more the body purges, the clearer gets the soul and the easier acts the spirit."

One of the stories I heard at the lunch table was of the patient who, purging with yawar panga, vomited up the residue of a codeine-laced cough syrup he had drunk eighteen years earlier, a residue that had formed a basis for his chemical dependence on cocaine. It was then I began to understand one of the primary differences between Western and Amazonian medicine: often a physician will attack disease *intrusively*, with medication or a knife, whereas a curandero will work *extrusively*, seeking to draw disease out of the patient's body.

To purge, at least in my case, was going to fling open the lid of Pandora's box. I didn't know this when the little Dixie cup, half-filled with the bright emerald juice of yawar panga, was set before me. If I'd known, I still would have drunk, but maybe I would have worried less about my sanity as the process went along. But Susana was seated beside me, and in her face came flashes of love sufficient to follow into the underworld. So when we raised the cups to our lips, I drank without hesitation.

The liquid ran down into my empty stomach and coiled up there like a snake of unknown potency. Smoke was blown on us. Perfume. An icaro accompanied by the whishing shake of a shacapa.

Then a pitcher of water was set before me. "Drink it all," I was told. "The more you can drink, the easier it will be on you."

At the moment, I felt okay. No nausea, no desire to vomit. Forcing myself to drink a liter, I heard Susana begin to purge beside me. Taking a deep breath, I put down the rest of the pitcher.

Refilling it, they told me to drink another.

My god, how much water could my body take?

Then my stomach took over. It felt like drowning in reverse. I saw the phosphorescent green remnants of the nasty cold I had been hosting for a couple of weeks floating in the bucket. The remains of my lunch. The bucket rapidly filled as I drank and vomited, drank and vomited. Caught in the coil of the plant, it seemed anything that could be ejected, was.

In the hours of that purgatory, I came to appreciate the stomach as the center of the human being. Lord of all it surveys. Hands, arms, legs, head, and brain all mere appendages of the central organ. Every muscle of the body at its disposal. Master Stomach threw me, its subject, into yogic postures of abject surrender until I could drink and empty no more.

Staggering home, still clutching our buckets, we fell into beds in separate rooms. Like a near-drowned man cast up on a beach, I finally coughed up thick, white mucus from the very limit of my entrails, and I fell into exhausted sleep.

I would like to say I awoke in the morning feeling like a new man, but I didn't. I did smell like a dead fish, however, and it was certain all the linen on my bed needed to be changed.

Wandering into the garden in my pajama bottoms, I approached the yawar panga vine and stood caressing its fat, heart-shaped leaves. Rust-colored veins fanned out across the face of the leaf, containing the "blood" that gives it its name in Quechua. Plucking a leaf, I opened one. A minuscule bright red droplet formed.

Blood. I had drunk its blood, then, and been given mild visions I could barely remember. . . . Susana appeared outside the door of our house, a cup of tea in her hand, looking bright and sunny.

"Hey! How are you feeling this morning? Renewed?"

Crushing the leaf in my hands, I put it to my nose. Inhaling, my stomach roiled, and I felt the presence of the vine still within me.

"No, not exactly. I feel more like . . . dislodged."

Rubbing shoulders with a number of shamans of different specialties at Takiwasi, we caught glimpses of the inner workings of their minds, the hybrid cosmologies these men of the jungle had evolved in the face of Christianity and technology. Cosmology is key to understanding men for whom the world is filled with spirits, alive in all its dimensions. And it is key to understanding how they heal. Healing comes from the successful reembedding of the patient into the sacred.

Don Ignacio was a *perfumero* and *tobaccero,* a healer who worked with the spirits of water. A powerful old man, he had the aspect of a wild, canny ape escaped from the jungle wearing human clothes. Buttonholing me one day in the hallway, he made me sit while he read my pulse. Instead of looking at his watch and keeping count, he seemed to tune in and listen to the flow in my body.

Looking at me with a grave expression, he said, "You suffer from *nerviosismo,*" and he went on to give a list of symptoms. Don Ignacio's Spanish came half-macerated from his heavy jaw, but I got the gist.

The following day I showed up where the little river called Shilcayo flows behind Takiwasi after its journey through the jungle above. There, under the supervision of Don Ignacio, a retired French secret service agent and I drank tonics of four medicinal plants: llantén, malva, lancetilla, and pampa orégano, to which was added at the last moment a more spirited concoction of Agua de Florida and thimolina, shavings of alcanfor, and Taboo. The perfume, that is.

Stuck within the prejudices of a Victorian Englishman, I leaned over to Don Ignacio's assistant, Jose, and asked, half-jokingly, "And why are we drinking perfume?"

"It takes out negative energies," he replied. "And it gives you protection."

At the last moment, Don Ignacio added tobacco to my drink. Tobacco I knew was used to treat addiction . . . and to open the mind.

Drinking the concoctions down, we paced about, and then we went to the river. Don Ignacio perched on a rock, and I, as per instructions, submerged myself in the water, gripping the stones of the riverbed to hold myself under as long as possible. Fish came to nibble at me.

Above the surface Don Ignacio commenced his icaro. Bobbing up and down to take in air, I heard him call to Jesucristo and the waters of the river to give me strength, to heal my nervousness. But who were Tia Robertina and Tio Pedro Forté?

The longer I spent in the river, the better I felt. Don Ignacio then called me out and sent me above, where Jose massaged me with a mixture of tobacco and perfume. As he did so, I asked him the identity of the aunt and uncle Don Ignacio had called to.

"Bueno, they are a couple, a *yacuruna* and *sirena* who live in the water and work with Don Ignacio."

Shivers ran through my body. Don Ignacio was calling on merpeople to heal me.

"He also works with a boa of the waters, a *yacumama*," Jose added. "The boa's phlegm enters your body and cleans it."

Don Ignacio reappeared to continue our treatment. Taking a silver crucifix from around his neck, he made me run in place while he sang and beat me on the head with it. Opening his massive jaws, he clamped down on the crown of my head with his teeth and blew out a thick cloud of tobacco smoke. Then he took a swig of Agua de Florida and drenched me.

"Fuerza!!!" he roared. "Strength!" "Look at me! I am an old man, but I am strong!" he said. "Who am I?" he demanded. He beat me some more with the crucifix and blew more smoke on the crown of my head. "Who am I?" he repeated.

Finally I saw it. The submersions at the river, the prayers . . .

"John the Baptist."

He grunted and nodded his head. I was off the hook.

Some days later, I asked him, "Don Ignacio, what happens when we die?"

"Bueno," he said, sitting beside me with the confidential air of someone about to reveal a very profound secret. I prepared myself for some esoteric jungle lore about the cosmic serpent or the Pachamama.

"When we die, we go to a place where there are two doors. One of them is locked and narrow to enter, but the other is always wide open. There we encounter San Pedro, who has the keys to the closed door, the one that leads into heaven. San Pedro has a book in front of him, in which is written all of our good and bad deeds during our lives. He consults the book to see if we are worthy to enter into heaven or not. . . ."

I felt like I had cut and slashed my way into deepest jungle, only to find a tympanum from above the doorway of a medieval cathedral, perfectly preserved in a curandero's head.

Although Don Ignacio had incorporated Christianity into his cosmovision, technology remained an utter unknown. He still responded courteously to machines assuming that a spirit was speaking from inside (of course, he may be right). He also displayed the same total indifference to images on a television as do cats and dogs.

The ayahuasquero Don Lucho, on the other hand, watched the Discovery Channel to learn more about the animals he saw in his visions. He also enjoyed Jackie Chan kung fu movies.

Oh yes, the treatment for my nervousness worked. Previous to Don Ignacio's submerging me in the river with the yacuruna and sirena, I had to wear shirts of light fabric and dark color because of the stains that would appear beneath my armpits in social situations. After the treatment, those symptoms completely vanished.

Walter Cuñachi seemed to follow the progress of the sun, his wicker armchair shifting from porch to porch as the angles of shade lengthened and diminished during the day. I would come upon him, loosely holding his staff, with its alternating rings of light and dark, between his legs, staring at darkness from behind his amber glasses, left facing whatever angle his son had placed him in.

A member of the Aguaruna tribe in which the women play the healing role, Walter had broken with tradition in that he had been trained as a curandero by his wife and he now led purges among the men of his tribe. Joking about his walking into posts, he entered the *maloca*—an open-air structure with a thatched roof—led by his son, and he took a seat before us, a huge vat of warm dark liquid beside him.

The vat contained *purgahuasca,* a dilute form of ayahuasca prepared with little or none of the magic leaves of the chacruna tree. The work of the evening was the opposite of ascending the shaman's world tree. We were going down into its roots instead, to drink the dark liquid and vomit for as long as we could sustain the process.

But in the face of our coming ordeal, Walter was gentle and welcoming. We had set up our bedrolls to sleep after the session, and he invited us to share our dreams with him and go down to the river to bathe before breakfast. He showed us scars on his legs and told us how he had used forest medicine to heal wounds that the doctors in town wanted to amputate for.

Walter's invitation to share our dreams confirmed my hunch that besides physical cleansing, the process of purgation was intended to reach to subconscious material in the psyche. For curanderos, physical illness begins first in the spirit, and vomiting is not, as it is for Western medicine, a mere side effect of physiological toxicity. It is a cleansing of body, mind, and spirit.

We received *sopladas*—the blowing of tobacco smoke like a fumigating agent down the spinal column, through the channel of the cupped hands to the heart, and upon our feet—to cleanse the body. We then approached the vat and scooped out bowlfuls of the dark liquid. Taking our seats on low benches, with buckets at hand, we began to drain the warm contents of our bowls.

Soon I was vomiting, tears streaming down my face, dazed like a little boy that had just been punched by the schoolyard bully and with the same sense of inexplicable injustice as a result. My stomach tensed like a trampoline. Reduced to delicately sipping the dark, acrid water in order to not toss it back up instantly, I tried to keep a balance between absorbing the medicine and vomiting it back out.

Finally, I was exhausted. Leaving my bucket on the splattered floor, I lay down to sleep. Half dreaming, I began to see the energies of a psychological complex dancing before me. But this time I recognized its source *in* my body. My shadow, fueled by subconscious energies I had been incapable of owning, was putting on a show.

Rolling on to my back, the *mareación** heightened. A scene played before my eyes: Susana in conversation with other men. A spirit of vigilance and interrogation started up in my breast. Scrutinizing her every move, my chest tightened with a will to project control.

What is going on here? I wondered. *I know what jealousy is. Why am I being shown this?* But then I noticed some strange interstitial vibratory thing . . . I saw it; moving with incredible velocity, a gray blur, back and forth between the figures.

Halting the scene as if I were a projectionist in a movie theater, the figures froze. Speaking into this suddenly empty, cavernous space projected by my own mind, I called out to the subliminal image: "Who are you?"

Out of the collage stepped a figure, and he had horns.

This is my shadow?

Pan, the Greek god, the shepherd trickster, stood grinning at me: the bridge between the sexuality of beasts and men, the frolicker on the margins between cultivation and wildness.

The whole, immense joke was unveiled. I faced my own emanation. Squarely. There was no denying it. And had he been giving me a run for my money!

I wagged my finger at him. "Oh, no you don't. You will *not* be playing these tricks on me without my permission."

The purga having brought my own projections before me in the form of a bucolic Greek god, there was nothing for it but to laugh. I dissolved into laughter from deep in my belly, halfway between weeping for relief and sheer hilarity. The incalculable merriment and strangeness of it all . . .

---

*The rise in psychotropic effect after ingestion of a plant.

Stirred to life in the dark of the early morning, we went down to the river, where Walter's son blew its water over our heads and feet, and we submerged ourselves in the Shilcayo's satin current, letting the river carry away the residues of the evening.

I was slowly making the acquaintance of another shaman as well, although at that stage only by reputation. I first saw Juan Flores Salazar in a photo, wearing a crown of brilliant feathers, regarding the camera with a half-smile on his lips and an innate regality in his bearing. The photo was mounted on a wall along with images of other curanderos who had worked at Takiwasi.

An Asháninca Indian, Flores had a serious mystique among the therapeutic team at the center, both for being one of the principal teachers of Mabit's, and for the mastery he demonstrates in directing the spirits of the plants. He had once shown this mastery in a remarkable experiment arranged by the anthropologist Jeremy Narby.

Narby brought three molecular biologists to Flores's center for traditional medicine, Mayantuyacu, to see whether, in sessions with ayahuasca, they could "obtain biomolecular information" in their fields of research. In a session orchestrated by Flores, the information came, but not through the ordinary "objective" scientific approach. For one participant it came through metamorphosis into the phenomenon she was studying: "The American biologist, who normally worked on deciphering the human genome, said she saw a chromosome from the perspective of a protein flying above a long strand of DNA. She saw DNA sequences known as 'CpG islands,' which she had been puzzling over at work. . . . She saw they were structurally distinct from the surrounding DNA and that this structural difference allowed them to be easily accessed and therefore to serve as 'landing pads' for transcription proteins."[8] These were ideas that had never crossed her mind, and she returned to her laboratory to verify the hypothesis. The two other scientists "spoke" with voices who offered counsel and instruction.

In interviews conducted four months afterward in their respective laboratories, the three biologists all agreed they had received information about their paths of research. The two female biologists also reported "contact with 'plant teachers,' which they experienced as independent entities," an experience that "shifted their way of understanding reality." The third biologist, a male, stated that "all the things he saw and learned in his visions were somehow already in his mind, but that ayahuasca had helped him see into his mind and put them together."[9] In other words, with him the plant took a more maieutic approach.

Lest this study sound too far-fetched for serious consideration, it is worthwhile to recall how the structure of the benzene molecule came to Kekulé through a similar process of human effort bearing fruit through visionary revelation: dozing off before a fire, the German chemist dreamed of a snake with a tail in its mouth arising from the flames, which he interpreted as meaning that the structure was a closed carbon ring.

All three research scientists expressed great respect for Juan's skill and knowledge; he had been able to orient them so quickly to the realm of visions *and* facilitate their extraction of useful scientific knowledge from the visionary state.

Over time, as the purges progressed, I began to wonder if I was showing the signs of an impending breakdown: uncontrollably swinging moods, chronic bad judgment, and emotional impairment. And to complicate the picture more, the "reality principle" was of little value in the realms of perception opened by the plants. Returning from an ayahuasca session held in the jungle, playing the amateur naturalist, I asked participants if they had seen any animals that evening.

Regarding me carefully, they asked, "Inside the maloca, or outside?"
"Both."

They started talking about the birds they had seen flying around the room in the pitch darkness of the night, animals I had been too busy being transformed into a jaguar to notice. I was puzzled until they called them protectors. Each shaman has spirit birds that protect them and the room during a ceremony, I learned. I suddenly felt dense.

"I meant literal physical animals," I amended.

"Then why did you say both inside and outside the maloca?" they responded, and I realized they possessed distinctions in language that I did not have. And they were seeing things I was not yet seeing.

And the culture was not doing its bit to help me sort out realities.

Teetering home from a purge with Rosa Sisa, I encountered our neighbor Alberto, one of the living exemplars of how this medicine permeates the culture, how in working with the plants we were simultaneously entering an underlying universe of folklore.

"It's good to do your purges as a young man," he told me approvingly. "It makes you strong in old age."

Sitting on his porch, I listened as he launched into a description of the powers of the shamans of old.

"It was with the *sapo,* the toad, that they worked. When they had an enemy, they imbued the toad with venom and would set it beneath a stone. When their enemy came walking along he would jar the stone and the toad would spit saliva in his eyes and kill him."

In my condition, Alberto began looking like a large toad himself. "But those were in the old days. Shamans aren't as powerful now as they used to be," he reassured me.

But he gave me the remedy, just in case a toad should be lurking nearby. I couldn't for the life of me remember the details.

Then there was the day we consulted Alberto's wife, a woman habitually dressed in black, about the bats in our house, the *vampiros,* who would shoot through in dark clawish blurs and vanish again back out into the night. I like bats, but Susana was concerned.

Fixing us with a haunted look, Alberto's wife said, "Oh, that's the *señora* who used to own the house. She used to transform into a vampire. Now that she's dead she still flies around at night."

The night the dreams came I was in the living room sleeping beneath the mural, a reproduction of an image remaining from the Mochica people, one of the high civilizations that had waxed and waned long before the coming of the Spaniards. In the mural two shamans, high priests, sailed like astronauts upon the back of a geometric field that was a serpent as long and spangled as the Milky Way, while sipping with straws from a cauldron of San Pedro.

Bursting into the room, Susana cried out, "Oh my god, Robert, did I just have a dream." I was instantly awake. Something strong was moving in our shaman's house.

Sitting beside me, she related her dream to me.

She had been visited by the green man, in the character of a peculiar little gardener who worked in Takiwasi. Always going about barefooted, with a machete in his hand and plants on his back, he had the stature and movements of a hobbit and words few and garbled in pronunciation and meaning. The perfect magician's assistant, he attended Jacques Mabit during his periods of fasting in the jungle with medicinal plants.

In her dream she too had been fasting in the jungle in a hut, drinking the plants. The little gardener came and in the form of a whirlwind raging through the trees, a howling of insects and monkeys, wild cats and devouring vines, laid siege to her. Throwing her weight against the door, she struggled to keep him out as the wood buckled and cracked, but finally the door burst in, obliterated, the force exploding her self and projecting her into outer space where she saw herself in a dark cosmos full of stars.

Waking in her bed, light as a feather, she jumped out and went to find me where I slept in the living room and realized, with her body become so subtle, she could fly. Waking me up, she cried out, "Robert, I can fly, I can fly!" while jumping around the living room. Grabbing her shoulders, I held her down, crying, "Why are you doing this? Why are you doing this?" Overcoming her shock and fear of no-self, she looked through the window and felt the desire to fly outside, but I held her to the ground.

Waking anew, she saw it had been a dream within a dream, a dream more real than real, and she again got up to find me where I slept. As she finished her account, I thought: it's the plants. The plants are becoming invasive, bursting into our psyches, their roots penetrating our unconscious. Suddenly I was afraid of what their inexorable progress would next reveal. Susana went back to bed, but not before she had cast the spell of dream over me.

Turning over, I went back to sleep.

I felt a wind tugging my garments, and then a rolling motion of a palanquin beneath me. Through an obscure light I saw figures moving alongside, some mounted and near at hand, but most moving on foot in a gray mass around me. The closest was a knight through whose travel-stained cloak gleamed the pale silver handle of his broadsword. Turning in his saddle, he revealed a white cross upon his back. The dark mass on foot was almost entirely of children, marching silently, their garments twisted about like leaves in the chill wind. The terrain was gentle, the Roman road wide and smooth. Looking to the east, I saw the outline of a castle jutting up into the pale blue sky upon the distant limestone mounts. It was early morning and the sun was rising.

Color began to spill across the army. I turned and saw a long column of children winding from the far horizon, spilling over the borders of the road and trampling through the meadows and woods. The gemstone the knight wore on his finger, the breath of his horse freezing in the cold air, the red hair of one of the apprentice boys, a green embroidered cloak worn by a girl of noble birth, and the purple and gold of the oriflamme bobbing in front of the army, all were suddenly visible.

The entire army wore crude emblems of white crosses sewn upon their backs.

I knew myself. I was Stephen de Cloyes, the boy prophet whose career I had once pursued across Europe and Africa. This was the march to Marseille, where I had prophesied that the Mediterranean Sea would part, allowing us to walk to the Holy Land and retake Jerusalem from the Saracens.

The landscape changed. Rain was falling. The road was churning mud. The children stumbled with fatigue, their faces thin and strained with hunger. The clothing of my palanquin bearers was tattered. Mud caked everything. Dark forms of children lay collapsed alongside the road.

The road became mountainous, the rain torrential, the way too narrow for the palanquin to pass. The army vanished, and my palanquin lay pitched over in the mud. Hearing screams of men and horses and the clashing of arms nearby, I pulled myself up upon a ledge at a sharp bend in the road and gazed down into a burning landscape.

Through the billowing smoke I saw a village, and then the figures of children with crosses upon their cloaks, milling about with panicked animals and peasants, pursued by mounted figures with round shields and curved swords, their white robes and turbans incongruous in the wooded landscape. One of the Saracens struck down a fleeing figure, and the child fell and remained still, his body a dark stain upon the ground. A terrible rumble of charging horses filled the air.

Then I felt my pilgrim's staff in my hand and smelling a sea breeze, I knew I was back in Marseille.

The dark sea murmured with the sound of a multitude of voices, as if within a cavernous chamber. Gazing into the darkness I saw something glimmering within. Seized by recognition profound and total, before I could form words in my mind, I was dashing for the seashore.

A little way down the rocky shore I halted. A city of light and weightlessness, of which the cathedrals I had known were merely crude echoes, emerged out of the darkness, striking my eyes like a newly risen sun. It was the Jerusalem we sought, but now I saw that we, I, had been mistaken. This was not the earthly city of terrestrial stone over which the sun set and the moon rose, through whose paving stones the first Crusader army had loosed a river of Muslim blood.

The Jerusalem we sought was this heavenly city of celestial stone, where the crude lights of the sky were superseded by the radiance of the Lamb of God, and the inhabitants dwelt in unimaginable bliss, their bodies transfigured and their lips singing the praises of the maw of light that had swallowed them like a whale.

Standing before the ocean in a daze, I saw in the depths the thing I had been seeking since I first knew my eyes and ears, catching intimations of its glory in earthly stone, wood, sound, and living flesh. The celestial city was my true home, and I knew I could no longer live without it.

When my senses returned from the golden twilight, I found myself surrounded by children of the army, now scavengers and beggars. Many were maimed by war, and had become its orphans. All of them gazed as well into the depths of the water.

One of the minor prophets, with blue eyes and long golden hair, his body unmarked by war, stepped forward. Grabbing my arm, he fixed his gaze in mine and said, "Give us the city of light." Making a sweeping gesture, he added, "Take whatever else you want, but leave the heavenly city." Looking around me, I saw holy relics encased in gold, icons, illuminated manuscripts bound in jeweled metalwork, silver crucifixes, and then crowns studded with gems, robes of Tyrian purple, swords, chalices, and tapestries. But none found a place in my heart. How could I renounce the home I had sought all my life?

Swinging my staff with deadly aim, I struck the minor prophet on the temple and felt the bone crush from the impact. The boy crumpled to the ground. Running the rest of the way to the seashore, I reached the water's edge and struck it with my staff, crying out, "In the name of God! For God's sake! Open! Allow me to pass!"

The sea rocked without opening. Looking at my hands, I saw they were coated with blood. Something struck me from behind, knocking me into the water. The light of the golden city went out.

The dream changed. No longer Stephen de Cloyes, I found myself in a land even more alien than medieval France.

I am a Gollum. A being long consumed by sin, emaciated as if with cancer, an outcast. I have returned to my hidden place to fondle my treasure: domestic objects, items inscribed with warm meanings for beings other than myself, symbols of home, of belonging. Of love.

A couch, a scroll, silverware. Records. A rug. A mug. My horde, never to be shown to the light.

I commited an unspeakable crime for them, and do not have the strength to leave them. Knowing I am damned unless I reveal my transgression, I choose to sleep as the guilt accumulates and consumes me in eternity.

Rising from the bottom of a thousand-foot well, I broke the surface of dream. Who was I? Stephen de Cloyes? This ancient creature from the depths? Or the flitting fellow of brief lifespan lying on his back in a room he couldn't even recognize? Still permeated by the gollum, I knocked on Susana's door, and sitting on the floor beside her bed with my head in my hands, I related my dream with the hollow voice of a medium.

Who was this gollum? Was it a crime from this life? A past life? Or was it a being from the dark regions of my addiction, still inhabiting my body's cellular memory? A thing that moved through the shadowy corners of jail cells and Tenderloin hotel rooms, alcohol-induced blackouts and the rush that follows the plunging of the needle into the vein? And, if so, had it finally been flushed out into the open?

I felt Susana's hand stroking my hair. "Congratulations, Robert," she said. "You're finally facing your shadow."

I went to consult with Jacques Mabit because, like Horatio, my faith still lay more in philosophy than in the language of the spirits of plants. I needed desperately to locate myself on a known map, even if I was in the empty, white spaces filled with smiling, spouting whales, two-headed men, and unicorns labeled terra incognita.

He received me into his office with a welcoming flourish and as we settled into a couple of chairs, he fixed me with a diagnostician's gaze. As I sketched the progress of my purges to him, Jacques suddenly reached up to a shelf above my head and took down a wooden dagger with a finely honed edge. Balancing the tip upon the fleshy part of his finger, he kept it there the entire time we spoke.

"Yes, it is sometimes baffling to discover, after fifteen or twenty years of work upon oneself, that what seemed to be resolved actually concealed unexplored vestiges," Jacques commented when I concluded.

"This can be explained, I believe, because there are three levels of self-knowledge, and most Western approaches only address the first and touch upon the second. The first is the psychic or mental level, and is more or less known, one can have a general view of it. The second level is linked to the complex of body and emotion, for which there are the various bioenergetic practices.

"And, there is a much less known third level that I call the deep somatic. It contains somatic inscriptions, *engrams,*" Jacques said, using a term from theories of memory function, "or the tracks of our whole life, of the deepest dynamic of our unconscious, and it appears to reach the cellular level. Indeed, this *soma* even contains the engrams or memories of ancestors, of the whole history of humanity, even of the cosmos. . . ."

The image of an astronaut that one of the patients had tacked up on his locker, floating in the starry void, came to me.

"People who experience plants of initiation, as you have, feel it, from their interior experience, as a very deep inscription, intracellular and perhaps nuclear, and these extremely buried stratums of the psyche come out."

"So all these years of Zen practice, aikido, periods of intense psychotherapy . . . they haven't been sufficient to really connect with and heal that old wound."

"The walking of the way of personal evolution, of self-knowledge, is compulsorily slow, Robert. And your experience of the purgas doesn't invalidate your previous work. On the contrary, that work allows you access to this deep somatic.

"I think what you've now discovered is that it is possible to resolve your problems on the level of your emotions and fears, and to successfully clear out the panorama of your life, without removing these inlaid engrams in the body."

"So I haven't been going psychotic lately. . . ."

"Well, if you stay at the level of these deep somatic memories, you would very possibly become mad or psychotic. This regression can only be temporary, because your life must be here and now, in this incarnation.

It is not really useful to get extraordinary experiences if nothing changes in our life. We are called on to *incarnate,*" Jacques said, his tone betraying his deep Catholic faith.

"And," he concluded, "one cannot penetrate into the deep somatic without first taking care of marking, as the Petit Poucet, the way back to the present."

A mysterious invitation to the deep jungle came in my final ceremony in the maloca at Takiwasi, at the juncture when we were preparing to leave the center to journey to Pucallpa in search of other curanderos with whom Susana could continue her studies. One of those healers was expecting us: Juan Flores, the shaman whose regal portrait had caught my eye in Takiwasi's hallway.

But the visionary invitation was presaged by a telling incident. Just before the ceremony, I requested *mapachos,* the cigarettes of black tobacco used by curanderos in their healing work, from one of the therapists. He walked to a white medicine cabinet with a red cross painted on its front and, to my surprise, opened it and took out a small bundle of cigarettes wrapped in plastic. He then handed them to me like a prescription drug.

Unwrapping them, I realized I had just been dispensed stale cigarettes. Looking at the blank expression of the therapist, I could see he had no consciousness of the vital power of the tobacco plant. At that moment, it dawned on me that Takiwasi still labored under the prescriptive mentality of Western medicine, and I would not find there the native intimacy with plants I was seeking. There also lurked an additional danger in approaching these powerful plants with a Western pharmaceutical mind-set: it could fling open Pandora's box, as I had just experienced, all too abruptly.

A maloca is the essential shelter of the jungle: an open-air structure with a finely woven thatched roof, watertight due to the ingenious natural design of the palm frond. Its form allows for the circulation of air in the still, humid jungle and it is as easily constructed as it is burnt down and abandoned.

The latticed walls of the maloca at Takiwasi contained us like a friendly spider's web, bejeweled with stars, from the aggressive buzzing and humming of the jungle outside.

The floor was covered with woven reed mats. Cushions were set out for each participant, a bucket beside each of them. Upon the posts hung images of the Virgin of Guadalupe, an icon of the crucifixion—El Señor de los Milagros—executed in what looked to be the Spanish style of Goya, and a baroque St. Michael slaying a dragon in the blue sky. Otherwise, the space was open and unadorned.

The patients of Takiwasi gradually gathered, dressed in white for the evening's work with ayahuasca. They were all men, from teenagers to old *campesinos,* workers of the land. Beside me sat a teenager who had come to Takiwasi to do a *dieta* in the forest, where he would follow a strict diet and take certain plants to clean his body and spirit. In the antique courtesy still maintained by the people of the country he addressed me as *usted* (sir) and had the grave, settled air of a much older man. That antique courtesy that was still maintained by the people of the country.

On the other side of the room sat the brilliant young Frenchman who aggressively disrupted the meditation session I led that evening. In the devotional Catholic environment of Peru, I had never bothered to explain that when Zen Buddhists bow, it is with the understanding the figure upon the altar is an expression of our own essential nature. We are, in effect, bowing to our awakened self. Now he sat in his habitual posture, head bowed like a vulture, before his inner torment of voices.

But it is not simply that he was an anarchist before God. His aggression arose from the fact I hadn't been walking my talk lately. The bullshit detector of drug addicts is very finely tuned, and as my purges had progressed the steadily hollowing sound of my speeches about meditation and awareness had been grating on his ears as much as they had on mine. The leaders, Rosa Giove and Jaime Torres, took their places at the head of the room, bottles of ayahuasca, Agua de Florida, and a juice of soaked and strained tobacco before them, along with other ritual implements such as the shacapa, which would beat in our ears like the sound of wings in the night.

One by one, the patients and I went forward to drink. *"Salud con todos"*—"Health with all"—we salute before drinking, the rest of the patients echoing back as a choir. Raising a cup of ayahuasca to the lips is a practice of transubstantiation. Within the thick, bitter fluid, capable of provoking instant vomiting, is the taste of the salvific power of the jungle, of evolution itself. That night I drank as if I were thirsty, the liquid flowing down my throat like honey. I regarded the cup in wonder.

Returning to my seat I clutched my prayer beads, willing myself to enjoy the beauty of the night before the onset of the visions. But a deep apprehension gripped my stomach. I found myself summoning my spirit guides with the urgency of one about to die. I would pass through the gates of horn—the ancient gate of true dreams—that night. I would have to, because the alternative was unthinkable.

Each ayahuasca ceremony at Takiwasi begins with an invocation of its teaching and purifying capacity. The sound of Rosa's voice gently arose over the buzzing hum of insects singing:

Madre Ayahuasca	Mother Ayahuasca
Llévame hasta el sol	Carry me toward the sun
De la savia de la tierra	From the nectar of the Earth
Hazme beber . . .	Make me drink . . .
Llévame contigo hacia el sol	Bring me with you toward the sun
Del sol interior hacia arriba	From the sun within toward the sky
Hacia arriba subiré, madre	Toward the sky I will rise, mother.
Úsame, háblame, enséñame	Use me, speak to me, teach me
Enséñame a ver . . .	Teach me to see . . .

A ver al Hombre dentro	To see the Man inside the
del hombre	man
A ver el Sol dentro y fuera	To see the Sun within and
del hombre	without the man
Enséñame a ver . . .	Teach me to see . . .
Usa mi cuerpo	Use my body
Hazme brillar	Make me shine
Con brillo de estrellas	With the light of the stars
Con calor del sol	With the heat of the sun
Con luz de luna	With the light of the moon
Y fuerza de tierra	And power of the Earth
Con luz de luna	With the light of the moon
Y calor de sol.	And the heat of the sun.
Madre ayahuasca	Mother ayahuasca
Llévame hacia el sol . . .	Carry me toward the sun . . .

Then Jaime sang, summoning spirits of healing and protection. Soon the maloca sat steeping in dense energy. The French boy thrashed about, constantly attended by Rosa. I sat in a revolving chamber of mirrors, seeing nothing but the confines of my self, amplified to the level of a custom-made Dantean hell. The other patients sat with heads bowed. The icaros went on to the dull flailing of the shacapa trying to cut through the darkness. Nothing moved. We were flies stuck in the bottom of a black lacquer bucket.

Finally after an eternity I was called forward to drink a second time. I tossed it down. Turning the cup about in my hands I contemplated my dosage. I knew that it was not enough, but self-medicating is not appropriate behavior. I returned the cup to Rosa and politely asked if I could drink more. She studied me in the darkness and, nodding her head, refilled the cup. I drank again. Now I was truly committed. I returned to my seat. Soon my head fell back to rest on the wall and my hands loosened their grip on the prayer beads.

Psychointegration, I had come to believe, is both the force and the goal underlying consciousness. It is what allows the little self to discover its true identity in what lies beyond it. Like gravity it contains the matter and temporality of mind, as well as providing the underlying, binding attraction of consciousness to the Self that lies beyond the narrow confines of the ego. That evening it came as a deity with a thousand faces and arms, a million eyes of spirits and gods speaking innumerable tongues, the free traversers of the depths of the mind. A voyage into the component beings that, assembled, make our character and psyche, dance in our neurosis, dream our processes, our births and our deaths.

Suddenly the spirit I encountered in the Barquinha church months before in Rio Branco, Brazil, hove into view in the darkness of the maloca. A blazing figurehead on the prow of my spirit boat cutting through the night. In a deep drift across the waters I became aware that my Nordic ancestors were assembling.

Ayahuasca literally means "vine of the dead" in the language of the Incas, and the taste of the presence of the dead is deeply familiar to a portion of our psyche we touch only rarely in deepest dream.

Now they were come indeed—those who knew how to see across the immensity of the ocean, bringing with them the Viking gift of sight, the virtue stored deep in my maternal lineage's genetic code. Half seeing their faces playing before me, half feeling the salt wind and wave upon my body, the paths of navigation suddenly lay bare, open. Ocean. Endless ocean. Brilliant, cold stars. I clutched the prow of the boat. I remembered.

Gazing like a drunken bear into a well, I then heard the sound of approaching wings—great wings, cutting across the water, mysterious and familiar at the same time. Then he came. Hovering over me, the dragon landed upon my head and closed his wings like a childhood blanket falling over my eyes. Settling into my cranium. Joining his vision to mine. The dragon I had fought so long and hard with, in the manner of St. George, in this center for the treatment of addiction. The serpent guarding his horde at the base of my brain stem, dark and poisonous, had returned—transformed as the joyous rider of the clouds to unite his vision with mine. No longer my enemy, he came to stabilize my spirit boat and to give me the far-sightedness I required as a helmsman.

"The dragon . . . the dragon . . . ," I muttered like a mantra, needing the sound to touch home in my body momentarily, aware I was journeying very deeply now.

Psychointegration released its hold and I passed out of the waters, though the presence of the dragon still lingered. I breathed into the night, trying to fix what I had just experienced in my mind. I felt not only the joy of a child at a wondrous thing; I intuited this vision as a benchmark in my struggle with my own patterns of addiction, as if they had been scooped out and replaced with a deeper presence.

After a spell I felt the arms of ayahuasca embracing me, enfolding me in a warm, fluid light and the circumference of her embrace became the walls of the womb. I was in the matrix of birth and rebirth, held. I rested.

The shamans came to visit much later in the session. The vision of the dragon having passed away, I sat like a pregnant woman in the early morning darkness, feeling the new life moving within me. Then the lilting, serpentine voice of Rosa, singing to the young man seated beside me, suddenly wound into me like an anaconda searching out deeper mysteries still, stirring something further down.

My body began to transform. My northern giant's bone structure began compacting into an indigenous skeletal frame. My skin darkened from white to brown, and I found I had been given indigenous ears to hear the sounds of this world and, what was better, the seeds of indigenous understanding were present in my mind. The strength of my Viking heritage was now serving as a bridge to pass over into being a native of this land, the land of Peru.

Now a smaller man with black hair, brown eyes, a sharp nose, and a different music sounding in his chest, I stared across the maloca and realized there was a presence there. Or presences.

"Bienvenidos," I heard. "Tu has hecho el trabajo y estas listo para venir a nosotros. Estas bienvenido a nuestra casa." "Welcome. You have done the work and are ready to come to us. You are welcome to our house." The voice came from outside, as if literally spoken to me.

The shamans of the deep jungle had come. I could not see any forms, but I knew them like I knew the smell of a wisteria vine. I felt very happy. Whatever this mysterious path was that I was being drawn into, it was opening further for me.

Ino Moxo were the final words lingering in my mind when the lights came on and the ceremony ended. I didn't know what they meant.

As the shock of listening to human conversation gradually subsided, I made an effort to circulate about the room. I found Miguel, shrunken and old, sitting wrapped in his blanket gazing off quietly into the darkness, his sixty some years of campesino existence and his struggle with alcohol and basic paste of cocaine weighing heavily on his frame. I sat beside him and asked how the session had gone for him.

"Muy buena," he replied, turning his face with its shrunken cheeks to me and addressing me formally with the assumption I was a doctor and not some scamp dharma bum from California.

I was content. Replete with visions. Jaime came and sat with us. I related my experiences of the evening to him. Mentioning that Ino Moxo had been the only name I had caught during the transmission from the jungle, I asked him who that was.

"Bueno, it's the Amawakan name for Manuel Cordova-Rios, the rubber tapper who was kidnapped as a boy and trained by Xumi, the great holder of shamanic lineage in the Amawakan tribe. But it's not really his name, so much as the spirit he was identified with. Ino Moxo is the *pantera negra,* the *yanapuma.*"

The words traversed the air with a chilling, feline gait. *Yanapuma.* The black panther spirit that had become one with Cordova-Rios. Had I been communing with the cat's human face that evening?

I had come to Takiwasi with the premise that addiction was at root a spiritual malady, cherishing the hope that the psychoactive and purgative plants in the indigenous pharmacopoeia could offer a royal road of recovery.

Just before our departure from Takiwasi, I spoke with Francisco, one of the addicts in treatment. When I asked him why he was there, he said grimly, "I had to taste things that were more human."

Francisco began using cocaine as a teenager. In Peru, the drug—a perversion of the medicinal, highly nutritional coca leaf—is plentiful, cheap, and potent. Five-gram bags sell for a mere twenty soles in Lima, which is around seven U.S. dollars. The recent marketing of "pasta," a paste made of the waste products of cocaine manufacture, has made the body- and spirit-wrenching high even more available on the streets.

Now in his mid-thirties, Francisco had passed eighteen years within the orbit of the cocaine experience, and he had been through several treatment programs before arriving at Takiwasi. "The first problem facing an addict is to develop the consciousness that the drug is bad. This is something that has to grow, and can take a long time," he commented. "All your horizons end with the drug. It's a terrible, strange pain. Nothing outside satisfies you."

As we sat facing each other on the floor of the chapel in Takiwasi, I could feel the rawness of the energy radiating from his tall, angular frame. Yet while not bothering to cover up the knife-edge of pain that sits in the center of his self, he spoke about his experience with remarkable humor.

A story he told me reminded me of the double curse upon addicts. The drug not only removes them from meaningful contact with the human society around them—life becomes a cycle of stealing, lying, and violence, as Francisco put it—but also from their own sense of humanity toward themselves. He related to me how after a six-month period enclosed in his parents' house, lost in paranoid fantasies so severe he only left to purchase more cocaine and could only sleep by taking rohypnol, a friend took him to a program called Paz y Bien—Peace and Wellness.

This program had many "houses" around Lima and had a reputation for uncompromising toughness. Addicts, once inside, were not allowed to leave until the relative who had signed the entry form reappeared and signed for their release. There was something attractive across the social spectrum in this arrangement—perhaps it was the punitive, quasi-monastic nature of the program, because both the very rich and very poor underwent the regime together. There was no counseling offered, no medications to ease the transition. Instead the inmates were broken down by physical abuse.

Francisco related to me how one day, after he had spent a time working in the kitchen, the director of his house appeared beside him and ordered him into the yard. There he was made to kneel, and when the entire community of approximately sixty people had assembled, he was beaten with kicks and blows by the various employees of the program. His offense was the suspicion that he had pilfered food. "But it didn't matter whether it was true or not. They would have found any excuse," he said, his eyes fixed on the floor.

After ten months of this coercive regime, Francisco's father returned. Francisco left the rehab facility "stronger" from the experience, he said, but profoundly depressed. In a visit to a psychologist afterward, he was found to be displaying the symptoms of post-traumatic stress disorder. Not many months later, the police discovered bodies buried in the yard at Paz y Bien, and thus the facility came to its cultic conclusion. Not long afterward Francisco confessed to his parents that he had started to use cocaine again.

After passing through other programs that attempted to replace his addiction with other addictions—television, antidepressants, Valium, neuroleptics, and so on—Francisco arrived at Takiwasi. In his first ceremony with ayahuasca he experienced the sky opening, and the voice of a woman told him, "You have to have patience, but your life is going to change completely." He then knew he had a future and he was part of that thing we call God. "I had peace for the first time since I knew I didn't have it," he said, laughing. "Since that day I've continued drinking and purging.

"I'm going to tell you something else. Not long after that first ceremony I had an experience in a session where I felt a spirit suddenly exit from the chakra in my forehead. It gathered in the darkness before me and began playing a scene from my childhood. It was as if I were watching television. In it I saw myself as a baby in the cradle, and hovering over me was a very black thing that I saw entering into my stomach and expanding up into my chest. I realized I had been possessed by a bad spirit, and that my work with the plants is to purge it out."

Work with ayahuasca and other plants was not a quick fix for Francisco, however. After several extended stays at Takiwasi, he returned home to Lima. After spending a month at his mother's bedside as she passed away, he returned to cocaine use again.

I asked him, "How do you control this impulse to seek solace in the drug? It doesn't seem to be controllable in the normal sense." I told him about Nancy Reagan's media brainchild, the slogan "Just Say No," as an example of the ordinary mentality about "controlling" the impulse to seek release in drugs. We broke into laughter.

"The treatment with ayahuasca is about integrating the dark part," he said. "It's impossible to control as a force outside yourself. Even if you succeed a little while, it will grow in force under the weight of that pain that doesn't leave you alone, and eventually you fall. You have to disintegrate first to see all the parts of yourself before you can reintegrate and become a new person again."

Francisco spends much of his time within the chapel at Takiwasi, in prayer. "I feel like I have a strong relationship with God because I don't have another way out," he said.

In his story I felt the uncontrollable hunger for self-transcendence lying at the core of addiction, an ache somehow akin to mystical yearning. It's as if addiction is the shadow cast in the world by our ultimate dependence on the nourishment of light, whether this need takes the form of the chemical process of photosynthesis, the warmth of a fire, the clarity of reason, or the ultimate glimpse of the light of the Godhead.

I went home and looked up a passage from a Jewish mystical text written right around the time of the missionary efforts of Jesus of Nazareth.

Violently agitated and trembling, I fell upon my face. In the vision I looked; and behold there was another habitation more spacious than the former, every entrance to which was open before me, erected in the midst of a vibrating flame. So greatly did it excel in all points, in glory, in magnificence, and in magnitude, that it is impossible to describe to you either the splendor or the extent of it. Its floor was on fire; above were lightnings and agitated stars, while its roof exhibited a blazing fire. Attentively I surveyed it, and saw that it contained an exalted throne; the appearance of which was like that of frost; while its circumference resembled the orb of the brilliant sun; and there was the voice of the cherubim. From underneath this mighty rivers of flaming fire issued.

To look upon it was impossible. One great in glory sat upon it: whose robe was brighter than the sun, and whiter than snow. No angel was capable of penetrating to view the face of Him. A fire was flaming around him. (Book of Enoch 14:13–23)

Surely, this was a vision of the sun that sustains us all. No wonder it casts such deep shadows in the human psyche. No wonder the world becomes unendurably barren after tasting that vibrating flame.

In the remaining days before our departure to Pucallpa, the enigma of my vision of the shamans of the deep jungle still remained to be unraveled.

It appeared I had fully stepped into the Cinema de Indio, a phenomenon that received its name during the rubber boom following World War I, when the rubber tappers invading the jungle encountered the native tribes and their ayahuasca brew. The visions that came when they drank inevitably reminded them of the new technology they had seen in the cities, where images from distant lands and times also miraculously appeared before them.

But the problem of how to interpret images seen inside the cinema kept turning over in my mind. The plant can magnify any number of aspects of the psyche, including material in the ego. In such cases, one could have a "vision" of the blissful consummation of a love interest arising out of loneliness, or become a jaguar as compensation for a feeling of powerlessness. I felt confident the vision of the dragon was a consequence of very concentrated internal work over the previous months, but what aspect of my psyche had the summons to the jungle arisen from? Was it sheer fantasy, or was someone out there really communicating with me?

So the next day I asked Jose Miguel, a young, thickly bearded psychologist on the staff who always radiated boyish warmth, about his own experience with visions. We had just pulled into Takiwasi with a load of goods to be distributed among the poorer employees there who had befriended Susana and me. He turned off the ignition, sat back, and thought about the question.

"I think when a vision is truly transpersonal, it comes out of the blue, as a surprise," he said. "And it is not related to personal history or the more obvious psychic contents."

"So the message of the shamans should be verifiable," I said.

"Of course," he answered.

5 THE SPIRIT OF MIST

The spirit of mist dwells with them in their receptacle; but it has a receptacle to itself; for its progress is in splendor, in light and in darkness, in winter and in summer. Its receptacle is bright, and an angel is in it.

THE BOOK OF ENOCH

Meeting a shaman naturally provokes a scrutinizing for gifts of power, or at least some evidence of otherworldly charisma. Standing on the sidewalk outside of our dingy hotel in Pucallpa, Juan Flores Salazar affected none.

A middle-aged man with short-cropped hair above a dark indigenous face with high cheekbones, he wore a frayed white shirt, old blue slacks, and scuffed black shoes. Addressing him as "Maestro," I shook his hand and found it hardened by a lifetime of work in the jungle. He smiled, revealing a row of tobacco-stained teeth, but his face remained set in the expression of deep stoicism the jungle gives to its inhabitants. He did

114

not make polite inquiries about our trip or lodgings, but stood, as silent and anonymous as anyone else we passed in this town bordering the Amazon rain forest. This was the Asháninca shaman who Susana and I had traveled across Peru to study with at Mayantuyacu, a four-hour journey outside the city.

As Susana chatted familiarly with Sandra, Juan's wife, he and I stood in the doorway out of the din of the motorized rickshaws, occasionally looking at each other and smiling cautiously. Finally it was decided we would go to a restaurant down by the waterfront of the river Ucayali. There we selected pieces of already broiled fish to be reheated on the brazier for our meal.

A very large, vigorous worm crawled about in a gourd set in the middle of the table, doing laps. I inquired what it was doing there and was told it lived in the trees and the Indians liked to eat them. Susana wrinkled her nose in disgust.

At dinner we gossiped about Takiwasi, and then, changing the subject, Susana and Sandra began chatting animatedly about the difficulties of taming the barbarians in their lives. They meant us. Juan and I glanced across at each other, and we laughed whenever the women discovered compelling parallels. I observed with envy that he was eating his fish with his fingers.

I've gotten too civilized, I thought, as I choked on a fish bone I hadn't been able to extract with my knife and fork. When I recovered, Sandra was relating intimate details of their courtship as Juan polished off his plate.

"I often can't tell if it's him or a plant that is talking," she commented during a pause, looking pointedly at her silent partner.

He smiled again.

I sat contemplating the possibility that this humble *indio* seated across from me was in disguise. Had he already introduced himself to me in the classic style of the shamans of the rain forest: through the Cinema de Indio? Among the features of this primitive (and therefore, I guess, original) cinema is telepathy. So apparent was this to early German researchers of the chemical constituents of ayahuasca that they named the first alkaloid they isolated telepathine, based on their conviction that what is now called harmine facilitated telepathic communication.

I suspected, therefore, that I already knew Juan. I believed it had been his spirit that had appeared to me during my final ceremony of ayahuasca at Takiwasi and had invited me to go study with him in the deep jungle.

But as we concluded arrangements to journey to Mayantuyacu in a few weeks, he still offered no hint of prior acquaintance. Watching him and Sandra climb into a motorized rickshaw and disappear down the dark streets, I remained puzzled.

Later that evening we took a walk in the outskirts of town where I encountered the creature, the one who keeps returning to my mind. Outside the tiny grid of the city center the sidewalks begin to pitch and lurch, suddenly dropping and ascending, and then the concrete ends. A medieval sprawl continues into the bare earth beyond, where its tradesmen and merchants, contrary to all gringo concepts of economic competition, flock together as birds of a feather.

A row of shops, all selling cheap *aguardiente,* the firewater of Latin America, with the same hand-scrawled price on a board outside the door, the same wares on display, and the same dissipated salesman, greet the eye. Down another block, bright yellow corpses of plucked chickens dangle from tabletops. Just around the corner, scribes sit in rows before their antique manual typewriters. The whole next section hosts the cobblers, who sit tap-tapping away at the soles of shoes, inside of boxes made of slatwood walls that close with a lid in the evening, as if they were a puppet show.

Barbers display a particularly ingenious setup. A barber can go solo with a briefcase and make his shop on any street corner, unpacking his mirror, combs, and shears, to give the cheapest haircut one could ever ask for, but those are strays. Real barbers have a stall they push to the spot where they want to do business that day, with a rack for all their implements and a seat for the customer. Choosing a certain empty lot, they congregate to pass the day in companionable shearing.

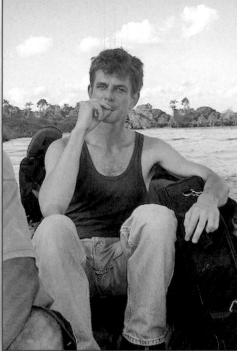

The author traveling upriver to Mayantuyacu, the healing center of master curandero Juan Flores Salazar.

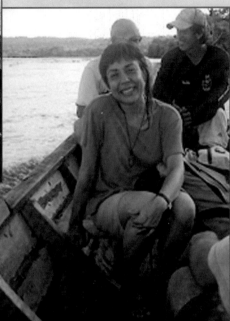

Susana ready to begin her fieldwork.

The wide expanse of the Pachitea River, the waterway leading to and from Mayantuyacu.

Juan Flores in ceremonial garments beckons from the mists. This photograph and the others on this page are courtesy of Fabrice Auguay.

The grounds and malocas with Shipibo designs at Mayantuyacu.

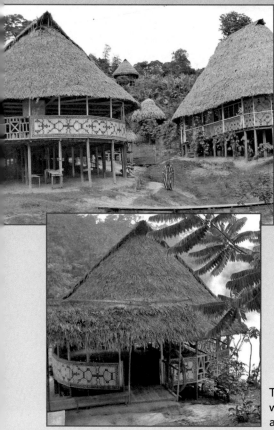

The central maloca at Mayantuyacu, where Juan conducts ceremonies and gives teachings.

Juan icarando with shacapa.

Juan prepares a fiery tonic from the root of the mucura plant.

The alchemical river of boiling water running through the heart of Mayantuyacu.

The first vision of Mayantuyacu.

The ayahuasca vine harvested from the jungle.

The ayahuasca vine is cut in preparation for cooking.

The preparation of ayahuasca.

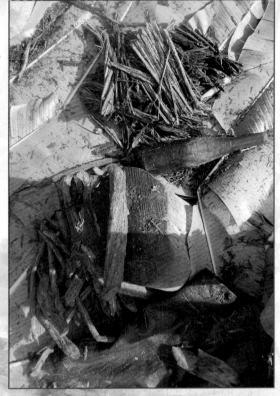

Ayahuasca boils
over an open fire.

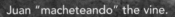

Juan "macheteando" the vine.

Juan's apprentice,
Brunswick, at work.

The vine of the came
renaco plant has healing
properties for bones and
connective tissue.

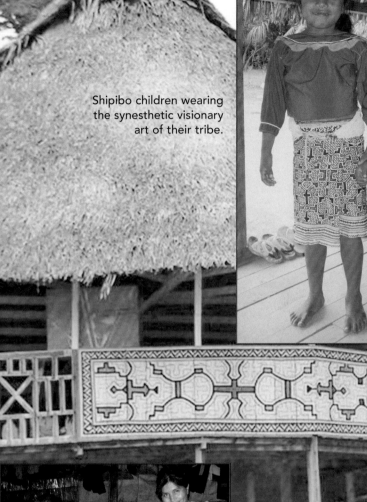

Shipibo children wearing the synesthetic visionary art of their tribe.

Two generations of Shipibo.

Shipibos working on song cloths.

Juan with shihuahuaco, a medicinal tree used in the apprenticeship of shamans.

Brunswick offers tobacco smoke to the came renaco prior to harvesting.

Susana and a local friend.

"The city for machines, the jungle for healing" — departing downriver from the healing center.

Also with their portable setups are the repairers and restorers of watches, the makers of keys, the fruit vendors, the lunch wagons with little pits of boiling oil, and finally, near the bottom of the food chain, are the waifs selling Chiclets and cigarettes from a small box strung around their neck, or offering you a shoe shine. Arriving at the bottom, the destitute approach your table dangling a baby from the hip or worn out after a lifetime of work with a machete and offer you a roll of toilet paper or a pack of pens. And finally comes the strange, almost electric shock of realizing the man in rags before you is begging to gnaw the bone on the plate that you just pushed away. Looking to the other side, you see a dog with a distended belly, eyeing the same bone.

Intermingled among the waterfront culture were the female members of the Shipibo tribe, a native people whose numerous villages line the shores of the Ucayali river that flows through Pucallpa. They were dressed in bright outfits with meticulously embroidered skirts to distinguish them from the non-natives. Whenever we were in a restaurant they would approach our table to sell us their fine handicrafts.

I saw the animal in front of a shop, illuminated in the lights of passing moto-cars, a silhouette tied to a white plastic stool. Approaching, I knelt down in the dirt, and it looked up at me with keenly searching eyes. Moving as close as its rope would permit, it carefully placed its hand upon my knee and began to speak. A language of high-pitched tones, accompanied by a startling range of expression, flowed over the wizened face of the medium-sized monkey. Its language was so close to human that I leaned forward and cocked my ear, as if I could catch some word or two that would make the specifics of its plaint comprehensible. I was sitting there fascinated when Susana appeared out of the night and crouched beside me.

"It's terrible seeing these creatures separated from their own kind. They're such social animals," she commented.

Taking its small, black hands in mine, I wondered at their leathery digits. We stroked its head, trying to comfort this poor animal now exposed to the pain of alienation, the shocks and buffets peculiar to our world. It tried to nestle its head into my knee.

The last glimpse I had of him, he was a silhouette again, dodging the mock kicks of children riding by on bicycles.

Holding hands, Susana and I walked back to the center of the town, talking about having a monkey as a pet. In the Plaza de Armas we saw a large crowd of people, tightly packed in a ring, looking in at some entertainment in the center. Lively music emerged from within.

Working her way to a gap between the shoulders, Susana peered in and whirled back to me, aghast. Taking my hand she said, "Let's go. There's a man with no arms or legs dancing around in there."

A surreal thrash dance, I thought. I looked at the ring of spectators: families with children, groups of young girls, couples, all gazing in with wonderment.

I thought again of the monkey.

During the final week we spent preparing to embark to Mayantuyacu, sitting alone in the dingy hotel room in Pucallpa, it came to me that there existed the nasty possibility that the Shipibo had hexed us.

My eyes fell on the turtle shell upon my desk. Painted with the radiating lines and mysterious figures that populate Shipibo art, it seemed to hold, encoded upon it and captured in the whirls of its energy patterns, an obvious and completely overlooked fact—a fact I rather needed to know now that I had fallen into a mysterious sickness—staring me mutely back in the face.

These patterns are written in the language of the plants, and are possibly *the perception of the world by a plant.* Today, however, few Shipibo possess the key to understanding this synesthetic ideographic language, for it arises from the perception, by shamans under the influence of ayahausca, of the energies underlying the visible forms of the world. But if there *are* any Sumirunas, shamans with full knowledge of this traditional art, they are now living deep in the jungle.

What makes you find yourself staring at these patterns in a semi-trance is the fact that they are translatable as music. The Shipibo creation myth[1] has it that in the beginning there was only darkness, in the midst of which dwelt a giant anaconda named *Ronín* who circles the Tree of Life—an image strongly evoking another serpentine twining: the DNA helix. This anaconda, reflecting back the images that she saw upon her beautiful skin, began to sing their geometric patterns, from which sprang the heavens, the earth, the celestial bodies, and all the creatures that inhabit these worlds. A world woven of the fabric of song was the result, and therefore even now each person and thing is imbued with their own distinct song pattern. By re-creating these patterns in their art, the Shipibo reconnect themselves to this original code.

Each pattern is an icaro, a song to heal, curse, cast spells, invite spirits, or open other worlds. The Shipibo heal by perceiving the energy fields in their patients and *singing* them back into harmony, something akin to how a physicist would correct an anomaly in a mathematical field.

The trouble began due to the fact that Juan Flores was one curandero among many in the region. Susana's study had already derailed at Takiwasi due to the unexpected loss of their mestizo curandero, and to put all our eggs in the one basket of Mayantuyacu seemed improvident. We therefore chose to take advantage of our time in Pucallpa to investigate the work of other shamans, particularly among the Shipibo.

The Shipibo curandero in question numbered among the urban shamans, belonging to the generations displaced from the jungle and the cycles of the life—animal, mineral, vegetable, and spiritual—that their ancestors knew. A small, plump man who peered out behind thick glasses, he had shown up at our hotel continuously smiling, like a ringleader in a circus about to introduce another act. He generously agreed to allow us to record the ayahuasca sessions that would be held at his daughter's house outside of the city, but the next morning he appeared unexpectedly in the lobby of the hotel with a request for a large advance upon the amount we had agreed to pay him.

Arriving the following evening at the curandero's home, we entered a space that had been cleared out in his daughter's living room/bedroom. The walls were covered with clothing hanging from nails. The sound of passing moto-cars, the rickshaws whose chainsaw engines fill the air of Pucallpa, penetrated the thin walls, mixing with the croaking of frogs in the river behind the house. A television blared in the next room. A baby with *susto*,* his eyes glassy from his encounters with the spirits of dead people, sat in shock on his mother's lap. A couple of "ayahuasca tourists," one from Japan and the other from Holland, sat waiting impatiently to drink for the first time. While one of the apprentices moved around arranging the room, I translated the shaman's instructions for the tourists. This included the price of the session. A soplada of tobacco, if they needed to be purified during the ceremony, would cost them an additional twenty soles in the ayahuasca tourist economy of Pucallpa.

Susana appeared beside me. "Come look at this," she said.

We went into the next room where the large-screen television dominated the living quarters. Hung on the wall was a seven-foot-long jaguar hide, the skull of its former occupant sitting on the floor before it. I caught a whiff of rotten flesh. Following us in, the shaman took the dried and shriveled paws of the cat out of a bag and set them before us. I turned them about in my hands as Susana admired the hide. The presence of the magnificent cat was still tangible, but its fragments made it seem implausible to my senses, like a badly handled museum specimen. Letting drop that he would sell the entire set of remains for two hundred soles, the shaman described how in a camp far down the river Ucayali they had accidentally surprised it, causing it to turn on them.

"Unfortunately, we had to shoot it," he said, putting on a long face, sensitive to our feelings as educated Westerners before the corpse of an endangered animal.

It occurred to me he was playing to his audience. He was lying.

Listening to the strangely Asiatic sounding polyphonic icaros of the

---

Sustos are a common feature of the landscape, particularly in urban shamanism. Dobkin de Rios describes them as "a common illness found throughout Peru and Latin America. This infirmity includes cases of profound alteration of metabolism, or nervous disorder. *Susto* is an intense psychic trauma provoked by an emotion of fear and includes lack of appetite and energy. *Susto* is caused by the loss of the sick person's soul."[2]

Shipibo, I lay down that evening and dozed off as Susana recorded the session. I completely relaxed my guard, and that was probably my mistake.

Waking in the early-morning darkness at the end of the ceremony, I found Susana packing her equipment. "Let's go," she said with suppressed urgency. I agreed. I had no desire to stay there any longer.

Immediately upon returning to the hotel, the illness struck. Night after night of wading through wisps of lingering sleep back and forth to the toilet followed. Finally, I dreamt of a landscape filled with water, water flowing in valleys, rising in vapors, falling lightly from the sky. Everywhere green, everything vibrant. Watching someone attempting to fetch something from the valley below, I called out to him, "Stop, you're going the wrong way!" Appearing on the next rise, he said to me, "I am a hydrologist. I know what I am doing." I knew instinctively it was Juan, going deep into the watershed to tramp through the resuscitating waters. "Wait!" I shouted to him. I ran in to find my shoes. But what shoes shall I wear? What flashlight shall I bring? Then I awoke to go evacuate muddy, fetid water, grateful I hadn't shat myself again.

The phone rang a couple mornings later, breaking into my reveries. It was Susana calling me from the Shipibo village of San Francisco down the river Ucayali from Pucallpa. There was only one phone in the village, above which was suspended a loudspeaker that was used to announce incoming calls to the inhabitants. Somehow Susana managed to get on it.

"I just met a guy . . . ," her excited voice announced over the phone. That meant she had encountered another shaman for her doctoral study.

Don Martín came walking through the trees to greet us the following morning, a very old man dressed in khaki, so thin his clothes seemed to provide needed bulk to his figure. His eyes glinted behind thick spectacles, and he wore a huge silver crucifix around his neck. He could have been an evangelist preacher man.

Don Martín had spoken very impressively with Susana about icaros the day previous, naming the various types, singing them in different tongues, and had read the pattern upon a Shipibo cloth and said, "This is the icaro of the white boa." He had also diagnosed her with a little black stone he held at the tip of his fingers and allowed to vibrate violently.

She needed *arkana*, he had told her, spiritual armor—sword, helmet, breastplate—to protect her because in her present condition anyone could come along and suck the healing songs that were in her right back out again and leave her worse off than before. And best of all, in a few aya- huasca sessions not only could he give her that protection, but he could set a subtle crown on her head that, like an antenna, would capture the icaros that the angels sing. . . .

Then he had proposed to do an ayahuasca session that very evening and get the work started. Susana had then called me. Did I want to come? Her excitement was contagious, but then in midconversation the line went dead. I didn't hear from her until she appeared at the hotel that evening.

"What happened to you?" I asked her.

"I kept trying to call you back but the line was busy the whole afternoon."

I called out to the guy at the reception desk and asked what had hap- pened to the phone that afternoon.

"Oh, it was off the hook," he said, shrugging.

"It's okay," she said. "I took it as a sign for me not to join the ceremony tonight, but he asked me for some money and said he's going to look at whatever is blocking the work with my thesis. Let's go back tomorrow. I want you to meet him."

So we returned. As our kamikaze driver barreled through villages and swerved to hit anything he could in the road, Susana related to me a story don Martín and his sons had told her.

Don Martín has drunk ayahuasca for most of his ninety years and had enjoyed good health the entire time. Then, a couple years ago, return- ing from a trip to Jerusalem, he suddenly fell ill and began to rapidly waste away. He went to the hospital and the doctors diagnosed a problem with his liver. They told him to lay off the ayahuasca. His lifelong consumption had probably damaged it and more drinking would only make things worse. He took to bed. Soon he couldn't walk and his sons were carrying him about on their backs. Finally, in desperation, he decided to consult ayahuasca. Seeing two witches of the village who had cast a powerful spell on him, he sent the curse boomeranging back at them.

"What happened to them?" I asked.

"They're in the graveyard now."

We were silent.

I watched the spry old man leading us back through his orchard to a compound with a large thatched roof structure in the center. Various little houses were arranged about. A radio blasted cumbias while his wife, dressed in Shipibo garments, moved about cooking over an open fire. It was hard to believe he had ever been at death's door.

Sitting upon a crude wooden bench, swatting mosquitoes, we faced the ayahuasquero.

"Did you see anything in the ayahuasca session last night about my work with icaros?" Susana immediately asked him.

He didn't reply, as if he didn't recognize what she was talking about. We chatted about other subjects. Don Martín talked a lot about Christ directing his work. He took out his black stone and vibrated it on his fingers for me. I then told him about my recurrent experiences with the spirit of the jaguar, of being transformed into the cat to the point of roaring and growling during sessions.

"I know that cat is a powerful healing spirit, a protector, but its energy tends to rampage through me and I want to develop a relationship with him so that he is my servant rather than an unpredictable ally. Besides, it's a little embarrassing to be making so much noise. . . ."

Don Martín's sons had gathered around by then and they all stood nodding their heads. Yes, the jaguar spirit is a powerful healing force. I told them how St. Francis is my ideal of the shaman, because he represents the man who has so completely tamed his animal nature that the birds of the air freely land on his shoulders and the animals of the earth gather peacefully at his feet.

Don Martín fixed his eyes on me and said out of the blue, "And how do you see me?"

It was an unexpected thrust. I studied him. His energy reminded me of practicing evangelicals—a bit stark, a little too much holiness, but that didn't have to be a bad thing.

"I'm new to this culture and I like to take my time in forming any opinions about things here. I'm still learning about this world of shamanism, but . . ." I studied him some moments more. There was something interesting about this old man. "There is something you have to offer that I would like to learn more about," I replied evasively. He and his sons all nodded their heads in approval. The silver crucifix around his neck rose and fell.

We discussed dates for future ayahuasca sessions. Having difficulty following the details of don Mártin's schedule, I walked away to fetch some money from my backpack to leave as an offering. Returning, I found him launched into his account of an ayahuasca session the previous night in which he had seen Susana being led by two angels to a throne of pure gold, and seating her upon it, they had set a crown upon her head. I took this to mean that they were opening her crown chakra to allow the heavenly songs to pour in but . . . it was all a bit confusing.

We made our reverences and left.

Susana was puzzled as I as we walked through the village.

"He kept changing his schedule on me. He said before he had to be in Lima a certain week but he just told me that he isn't going. And he said before that on Christmas Day he wasn't going to be here and now he is. And did you notice how when I first asked him if he had seen something in the ayahuasca session last night he didn't answer, and then he told me that whole vision right before we left?"

Finding a place to sit, we watched the life of the village. Loud rock 'n' roll poured out of one of the shacks with a corrugated tin roof. On the other side of the street, a Seventh-day Adventist church—the best structure in the village—was beginning its services. Shipibo in white shirts and slacks, Bibles in hand, were gathering on its steps. Little children ran up and asked if they could sing for us. Their voices were sweet and lilting, until they asked for money. A statue of a Shipibo in traditional garb fashioning pottery stood on the main corner, as if to memorialize a way of life already passing away.

What began as a conversation about future plans suddenly opened into a rift in the very foundation of our relationship. I was ready to catch a plane back to California. I was exhausted from the inner work at Takiwasi, I declared, and from living in a culture so alien to all I had known. I yearned for a time in the mountains, and to be with my community again. We entered into a very intense, quiet argument. We moved off to seek some privacy by the river, facing the possibility we might not make it together if we didn't find each other again. It was as if in a single morning we had become lost inside of a nebulous cloud. An hour later, as we sat in silent agony, a woman politely approached, asking us what we were doing in San Francisco and inviting us to come look at her handicrafts. We told her we had come to visit the curandero don Mártin.

"Él no es curandero, es brujo!"—"He's not a curandero, he's a warlock!" she spat out. "He killed my brother-in-law with witchcraft. He wanted the land next to his own, and when my brother-in-law wouldn't sell, Martín threatened him. Right after that, my brother-in-law fell sick and within a few days he was dead. Martín got the land. Whenever he gets drunk he brags about how he killed him."

Things suddenly began to fall into place. The big cross. All the talk about Jesus. The shifting stories and grand promises. Susana recalled how, during her visit the day before, she had tried on Shipibo garments at the invitation of don Martín and his wife, an invitation she had interpreted as a gesture of friendship. While don Martín's wife was helping her dress she suddenly felt the ayahuasquero's hand on the backside of her neck, as if fixing the upper part of the garment. His hand felt cold and in the wrong place.

We went back to the village and made discreet inquiries. The people grimaced and shook their heads. Whatever don Martín and his sons were doing, they had no friends there.

In a store with a few shelves of merchandise we sat with an asthmatic old crone who showed us her poor wares while lamenting her deteriorating health. Susana urged her to go to a clinic in Pucallpa, but where was she to find the money? Leaving, they embraced, and turning to me, the crone seized the opening and planted a bacteria-crawling kiss right on my lips. I walked down the road washing my mouth out with bottled water.

We caught the next car back to Pucallpa, chilled in our souls, but reunited. I decided to tough it out and stay in Peru with Susana.

Naïve psychonauts arriving in Peru seeking authentic shamans to help quench their thirst for authentic spiritual and ecological experience are the new foreign import ripe for exploitation. According to anthropologist Marlene Dobkin de Rios, there has been a recent appearance of unscrupulous tour operators (particularly in Iquitos) offering "shamanic services" in cohoots with "charlatans . . . without any special training, with little knowledge of disease process or biochemistry, and who are prone to use witchcraft plants (read, 'poisons') to ensure that their clients have a good trip. Moreover, the suggestibility properties of these substances . . . are, on occasion, used by some new ayahuasqueros to aid in the seduction of female participants. On occasion, madness or death has followed when the new shamans add plants, often in the nightshade family, which contain substances that are added to the mixture." According to Dobkin de Rios, there have been three recent deaths from ayahuasca ceremonies gone awry. It goes without saying that these businessmen in shamans' clothing "have never been apprentices, nor fasted or adhered to special diets employed by traditional healers" necessary for mastery of their crafts.[3] A pernicious side effect of this burgeoning industry of ayahuasca tourism is the disappearance of ayahuasca as a sustainable plant in the Amazon.

Brujería—witchcraft—is as well a serious issue in Peru, a constantly revolving door of hexes and counterspells and exorcisms. Descending one morning to heat my coffee for breakfast in our hotel in Pucallpa, I noticed the mother cat was missing her kitten.

"Where'd the little one go?"

"She was stolen." The cook was clearly heartbroken.

"Why would someone do that?" I asked her.

"It's because she's black. Black cats protect against sorcery."

Another morning, just before leaving Takiwasi, I was talking with our neighbor, a vigorous old man with bandy legs, whose carpentry shop began hammering away just after sunrise every day. He'd been a good neighbor, open-handed with us, and that morning I offered him a freshly ripened bunch of bananas taken from our garden.

"You're not going to eat them?" he asked me.

"No, we are beginning a diet of camalonga, and we can't take sugar or fruit with it," I replied, thinking such esoteric information would hardly be of interest to him. Camalonga is a plant whose golden spirit gives golden dreams, whose seeds, when steeped in a solution of yellow aniline, create a bitter, arsenic-laced potion used as a protection against black magic. We were were drinking this concoction in preparation for our journey to Pucallpa, brujería capital of Peru.

His face lit up. "Ah, yes, camalonga!" he declared. "I diet with it six times a year for a week!" Then he went on to explain to me how garlic and ajo sacha are also very useful in warding off sorcery.

What does this benevolent old carpenter need to protect himself from? I wondered. But then I remembered the unusual degree of knowledge of plants he had displayed while wandering around our shaman's garden, and I realized that perhaps carpentry was not the only trade he plied.

And then there is the ace in the hole of brujería, the *virote,* possibly the most virulent of all aboriginal technologies. The virote, quite simply, is a magic dart: a dart that many shamans master during their apprenticeships and use to kill, sicken, or drive rivals mad. They also employ them when they hire themselves out as hit men.

After some weeks spent living in the intense ecological competition of the jungle, where everything is feeding on everything else, one can begin to understand how such practices could arise in tribal cultures in constant warfare with one another, but it doesn't lessen the sense of evil in the tales one hears. For this reason, we learned that shamans who work in the light must be very, very conscientious about keeping their own spiritual houses in order. Virotes, like insects and disease, attack where one is weak.

We visited the famous painter Pablo Amaringo, whose work has come to define what, according to the French, is the New Amazonian style of painting, at his Usko-Ayar School in the outskirts of Pucallpa. Don Pablo is a small man with a trance-inducing voice and an unfailing gentility, from whom bursts forth visionary landscapes of incredible detail and subtlety, freely mixing highly evolved concepts from different spiritual traditions while remaining rooted in the world of Amazonian curanderismo.

Bringing in rolls of canvas, he unfurled his three most recent works before us. Meant to be read like books, they are something like the art of Tibetan tankas or medieval cathedrals, except that Don Pablo's cathedral is the forest, a sacred repository of untold worlds of knowledge.

"Each plant has its property. They made me see they are huge libraries, millions of libraries, millions and millions. Each plant is a library. When men destroy the jungle, they've burnt a library of books without even having been able to read them."

We lingered over the paintings, as if they were scrolls preserved from an ancient culture, admiring the technique and mastery of colors that evoked the living hues of the jungle. Like Shipibo art, the images were obviously seen from another eye than merely the physical.

"When you listen to the song of a spiritual being, an icaro, what a marvel!" Pablo said, pointing at one of the princely figures that inhabit his landscapes. "Frankly, what a marvel! With this song you could live for millions of years. No desire to eat. You don't want anything, you're so content. The first time I heard an icaro, I said to my master, 'I would like to live with this for the rest of my life.' Without it wouldn't be living. The contentment, happiness, I don't know how many other things, but how, how beautiful. Those are the icaros."

We asked him about the brujería practiced in Peru. "Let me tell you the story about the first time I was spiritually attacked," he began, and launched into a tale:

I was not born in Pucallpa. I was born in Tamanaco, lower down from here, and I lived there until I was ten years old and then I came here. I returned to Tamanaco when I was eighteen to visit my brother. The people saw that I had come back still young and welcomed me. Everything was very pleasant. I spent a month talking with folks, visiting.

One day I was passing through the village to where I lived, an hour and a half walk down the road, and a señor invited me to visit his house. "Come in and visit with me," he said, but the sun was already setting, disappearing into the trees, hiding itself. I was carrying a lot of fish, palometas, a very large and delicious fish. So I told him, "I cannot, Señor Santiago. I cannot. It's already getting dark and I have to walk another hour still. I'm afraid the snakes in the road will bite me. I cannot. So I will go, but another day I will visit with you." I said, "See you later!" and as I turned to go he sent the chonta, the virote, la aguja, at me. It was a needle of wood. He shot it in my neck, at the jugular vein, in order to kill me. But he missed, and it went into another part.

"Don Pablo, was it a literal arrow?"

"Yes, because one can see it. Those who know how to heal can see them. A doctor who has dieted well certainly can see them. But when someone has no training and is simple, he doesn't know."

Then in the middle of the night I awoke and shifted my body. I began to scream. It was like a needle was jabbing into me. I remained frozen. I couldn't move my neck. So my brother came in and rubbed my neck and said, "Maybe someone has done you a daño, brother. Someone has cast a spell on you."

I laughed and said, "You all live in ignorance all the time. When are you going to awake from this ignorance? This sleep in which you dream, ignorant people? How are they going to attack me here? Why? Who would do a daño to me? No, it's a shock from the air. I wasn't sleeping well and I twisted something."

Well, dawn came and when I tried to swallow I still felt pain. But

I didn't pay it any mind. Around one in the afternoon I couldn't drink water anymore. Then a very high fever began, and a burning around my head like the stinging of wasps.

I couldn't support this stinging around my head, and I felt I was approaching an abyss. I didn't know where it was going to take me. So I said to my brother, "Take me to the person you told me about, where I can get well again." It was already eight in the evening and they took me in a boat, one with oars, not a motor. They covered me up and took me down the river for two hours to the house of the doctor, the curandero, who was just coming into the port from his day's fishing. At exactly the moment we arrived, the curandero was tying up his boat.

My brother called out to him, "Can you help my brother who is sick? We don't know what is the matter with him."

And he called to me, taking me by the right arm. "Ah, someone has done a daño to you. Why? Come up to my house and I will give you a treatment." So we went up and they prepared themselves a meal. It was near midnight and they were all laughing, very relaxed. When they were done the curandero said, "Everyone to bed! I am going to do some healing. I am going to cure this boy."

I had a high fever, and I watched him from beneath the blankets. He took out his tobacco bag and pipe, like this one here, very large, and half filled it with tobacco and began to smoke. He smoked and swallowed, smoked and swallowed the smoke. Three times he did it, and then he let out a roar. It frightened me. It was something I had never seen before. What was going on here? Again he smoked, and again he roared and it was as if there was something in his mouth that was coming out. And he hit his head like this. Again he smoked, again the same thing.

Then he went to one of the corners of the room and blew smoke and there was a sound. Tchi chi chi, tchitchi chi chi. Little birds began flying about the room, but where did they come from? Then he did the same thing in another corner. Tchitchi chi chi, tchi chi chi tchi. And he did it again in the corner where I was, right here. I was watching. He came and blew and tchi chi chi tchichi chi. I was astonished. What were these invisible birds who when he came and blew smoke went flying through the air crying? I doubted my own eyes.

Then he came to me. "Where is the hurt?" he asked. "Where is the pain? Show me." And he touched me there, very slowly. "Ah yes, here it is." He lowered his mouth and I didn't know what he was going to do. Bite me? Then a long, thin tongue came out of his mouth and entered me there, making deep sucking sounds. Then he spat.

"Yes, there it is. It's out now. What is it? Let's see. Bring the lamp." They brought the lamp and there it was in his hand. A needle of cumaceva, the wood of cumaceva, very jagged, covered with blood and phlegm and I don't know what else. He took it up to his mouth and bit off the tip, like this, and blew it away. "Now we can see the dart!

"Now you can sleep peacefully," he said. "Move your head slowly, rotate it." I could move it again. The fever had left me too. I got ready to sleep, and he told me, "Now I am going to see who did you this daño." At five in the morning, while it was still dark, he said, "Pablo!"

"Yes, grandfather," I answered.

"I now know who did you this daño. It was Don Santiago. Before coming here, you passed by with a lot of fish in your hands and he invited you to go up to his house. But because it was already late, you didn't want to and you continued on your way. When you said good-bye and turned your head he tried to kill you. But he missed the vein. If he had hit it, you would have died in your bed."

That was the first time I realized that these things are real, but I thought later, No, I don't understand it, but it can't be like it appeared . . . *and I continued doubting.*

Just as *The Phantom Tollbooth* had appeared in my moment of need in the children's shelter, a map now fell into my hands: a tale whose hero's strange, winding path I could locate myself upon.

It came in the form of a tattered paperback copy of Gottfried Von Strassburg's version of *Tristan*, lying displayed on a street vendor's blanket amid comic books and Bible tracts. It leaped out at me, and I bought it for five soles, hardly suspecting that it contained a guide for slaying dragons. The tale is very old and part of the pre-Christian bardic repertoire of the Celts. Coming into the hands of the poets of of the Provençal courts of Eleanor of Aquitaine and her daughter, Marie of Champange, these tales were transformed into the courtly romances, which provided keys to journeys of inner transformation for masculine chivalric culture far outside the control of the medieval Church. Within this powerful medieval queen's strongly fortified walls also briefly flourished the Courts of Love, troubadour song, and the numerous heresies of spiritual purity then challenging the Church.

The story of Tristan and Isolde is now chiefly remembered for its love potion, which unites the lovers in an ecstatic and ultimately tragic fate. As I got drawn into the book, however, I saw the healing power of the tale lies in the initiatory death that Tristan undergoes when he first arrives in Ireland on his mission to bring Isolde back to Cornwall as his uncle Mark's bride.

As the tale goes, a dragon of terrible ferocity and destructiveness is ravaging the country of Ireland, and King Gurman issues an edict that any knight who slays the dragon will be given the hand of his daughter, Isolde, in marriage. Tristan, hearing about this state of affairs, naively decides to do the deed in lieu of King Mark and so win Isolde's hand for his king by right as well as by diplomacy.

But the battle is far harder than Tristan had expected. His horse is burnt and devoured beneath him, his shield is charred to cinders, and he himself is nearly consumed by fire. Finally, the dragon begins to flag and Tristan manages to thrust his sword down into its heart.

With the death of the dragon, Tristan, in a strange ecstasy, pries open its jaws, cuts out its tongue, and thrusts the severed organ beneath his armor against his bosom.

That old serpent, I thought, remembering John's Revelation. Trampled under the feet of victorious virgins, slain by good old St. George, and chained and cast into a bottomless pit by St. Michael. The bane of Beowulf, the creature whose blood Siegfried drank to understand the language of the birds, the Smaug whom Bilbo the thief outwits, the Shai-Hulud, whose drowning water Paul Atreides drinks to become the Kwisatz Haderach.

And yet, "Be wise as serpents and harmless as doves," Christ instructed his disciples.

As any shaman will tell you, there is great wisdom in the serpent, but to receive its blessing its energy must be mastered, *transformed through the body*, a mystery reflected in the old French tale in which *poison* is the same word as *potion*. It is medicine—medicine that kills and brings back to life.

The vine of the dead . . .

Akin to the functioning of ayahuasca, having seized the dragon's tongue, Tristan will now hear what it has to say across their different natures. The dragon's heart now united with his own the poison/potion of the dragon's blood begins to work upon him.

Staggering to a pure, shimmering pool of water fed by a burbling rill from above, he falls on his hands and knees and drinks. Then rolling over, he sinks into the water, armor and all, so that only his mouth and nose remain above the surface. Going into deep miraçao, he begins to integrate the power of the dragon, and he lies as if dead for a day and night, "for the cursed tongue which he had on him robbed him of his senses."[4] Tristan, caught in the tentacles of death and rebirth, has returned to the matrix of the womb.

Meanwhile, strange things are afoot. The king's steward encounters the slain dragon and Tristan's half-consumed horse. Believing Tristan dead, in true Falstaffian style he hacks away at the dead beast for a while and then rides back to the court, bragging loudly of his prowess, to claim the princess as his prize.

The princess, Isolde, and her handmaiden Brangane ride out to the site of the battle to investigate. There they find the corpse of the dragon and set off in different directions to seek its slayer. The princess Isolde, drawn by a vision of Tristan's shining armor—or his soul's radiance—discovers him lying in his watery grave/womb. She comes as the energy of the dragon transformed, the feminine aspect of Tristan's soul, to awaken him from his sleep.

In the remarkable way that such traditional tales reveal underlying patterns in our own lives, I saw how Susana had appeared as my Isolde the day I first held her hand and walked with her down the Market Street I had wandered as a boy, through that wasteland of the bottle and the needle.

That morning I had shown up to chauffeur her around town as she attended to the final paperwork for her Ph.D. study. She clambered into my old truck (the passenger door was stuck as usual) dressed in flowing garments of pink and purple, and we set out for the grave halls of academia. As we drove, we told each other children's stories about magic buses and the Aeroguatutú, a vehicle that resembles an egg and can fly and be transformed into a boat and be driven on roads, but it's so slow everyone honks at it. Thus its name: *aero* for "air," *gua* for "agua/water," and *tutú* for the "toot! toot!" of honking horns.

Meeting in a café later in the day, Susana stood up and studied herself in the mirror. "I look like such a hippie now," she said, and told me about her business suits and the cellular phone she had carried when she worked ten hours a day in drug abuse prevention programs in Chile.

The Indian restaurant we wanted to eat at lay far in the distance, and we had actually found a good parking space downtown. As we started off down Market Street somehow I offered her my hand and she took it and we just started to walk.

The territory of gleaming silver and glass of San Francisco's commercial district came to its abrupt end, and the long panorama of men and women hunched over their plastic begging bowls, scraggly animals, shopping carts, sleeping rolls, cardboard boxes, and bottles in brown paper bags stretched before us. Memories of my life there came swirling back, but that day I wasn't trapped in them.

Susana halted suddenly.

"Oh my god," she said, gesturing toward a man in a light jacket, with short hair and glasses, getting out of a vehicle across the street. "I worked with him in the prison where I did music therapy. He sang in the choir."

The guy was anyone in the streets. The close orbits between the worlds of prison and the streets hit me anew. My guard began to come up. "He's a really talented poet," she added. "He composed a rap song that he performed for the inmates and he, this introverted white guy, blew them away, including the black ones."

Half-concealing herself behind me, she said, "I think we should go. The prisoners aren't comfortable meeting people outside that they knew while inside."

We moved on and I relaxed. Learning to see the inhabitants of the street through her eyes, I saw the compassion in them. It was easier than I thought. I began telling her about my own adventures on those very pavements, and something of the desolation of it all. It was the humble voice of someone still working on his recovery.

"And how is it for you now?" she asked.

"Well, I'm walking down these same streets holding hands with a beautiful girl from Chile," I answered.

Flowing past the homeless who were warming themselves in the gritty San Francisco sunshine, the streets were changed. A beam of light penetrated deep into the cavern of lost souls, both within my own repository of memory and in those lying in their various stages of dying along the red bricks of Market Street.

All of these beings within me would have to be brought to the light to realize the depth of love Susana was stirring in me. It was no wonder I ended up drinking yawar panga at Takiwasi two months later.

But that day I was Tristan when he awakes, beholding three women gazing down upon him like the Celtic trinity of goddesses, naturally imagining himself arrived in heaven.

But even then he does not know he loves Isolde, or Isolde him.

As Tristan's tale continues, he brings Isolde across the waters from Ireland to Cornwall to marry King Mark. Becalmed upon their voyage, Tristan and Isolde call for a bottle of wine. Brangane, who had been entrusted with a love potion by Isolde's sorceress mother with instructions to administer it to King Mark and Isolde on their wedding night, has carelessly left the bottle sitting out and a servant girl serves it to them by accident. They drink and the sea is becalmed no more. A tremendous storm arises through which they sit feeding upon each other's eyes, unheeding of anything occurring around them.

This, I thought, is the true nature of psychoactive medicines.

The shamans of the Amazon, we now knew, sing a certain species of icaros, also intended to catalyze love, under the influence of another vine. As we were to hear Juan sing in ceremonies:

Palomita blanca, dónde estarás	Little white dove, where
túuu?	will you be?
Lejos de mí y lejos de míiii . . .	Far from me and far from me . . .
Dame tu pensamientos que yo	Give me your thoughts which
los guardé	I will keep
Y mis pensamientos serán para	And my thoughts will be
tiii. . . .	for you. . . .
Dame tu corazón, que yo	Give me your heart which
lo guardé	I will keep
Y mi corazón será para tiiii. . . .	And my heart will be for you. . . .
Cuando sale el sol te pondrás	When the sun sets you'll
a llorar	begin to cry
Llorarás porque, sin saber por	You will cry because, not
qué . . .	knowing why . . .

This is a gentle love song, filled with yearning and woven with magical spells. There is little harm in singing *huarmi* icaros, or songs that cast spells of precipitous love, Juan informed us a little disingenuously, because nothing is going to emerge that wasn't already there . . . and by the same token, if the enchantment works it's only temporary.

In the case of Tristan and Isolde, the effect of the love potion is not merely to make them infatuated with each other, but to catalyze the seeds pre-existing in their consciousness. It burns away the perceptual dross preventing them from seeing the depths of the bond that *already* is there, the dragon's blood having already awoken the deep memory of their love for each other.

What they discover is that marriage is the inevitable consequence of slaying the dragon: Tristan and Isolde are joined together in the *hieros gamos,* the sacred marriage. The rest of the tale lies in their struggle to reconcile the demands of the external world (Isolde marries King Mark anyway) with the far stronger bond that has been laid upon their fate as dictated by their encounter with the dragon.

What I didn't know at the time was that the cartography of the book was not just laying out the past, but was also foreshadowing the future. I could not know how desperate the battle with the dragon was going to be.

The journey to Mayantuyacu took us far out of Pucallpa to a little pueblo named Honoria on the edge of the Pachitea River. Honoria is a town that enjoys three hours of electricity a day and has a single antique computer whose Internet connection strains and wheezes to bring up an image from the world outside. Finishing our last Inca Kola on the veranda of one of the wooden structures that spring up like riparian growth along the water's edge, I asked Juan to stand before the river for a photo. He acquiesced, but as he faced the camera I sensed that the image would capture nothing because he had still not revealed anything of himself to us. We descended to a long canoe with an outboard engine, slung on our backpacks and computers, and set off upriver.

The Pachitea is wide and slow and muddy brown like all Amazonian rivers, the foliage along its shores punctuated by sections where the faces of mestizo children poke out from behind the trees. Little farmhouses on stilts suddenly appear, and their inhabitants, frozen in the postures they had adopted just before your coming, look at you. You look back almost embarrassed to be given such a glimpse into the book of their lives. Susana and I sat facing each other in the canoe, beaming.

Twenty minutes later the prow of the canoe was driven onto the shore and we clambered out to find that people from Mayantuyacu had hiked out to meet us and carry our baggage in. We ascended to a wooden shed with a plank gangway leading up out of the mass of rooting pigs and the mud. The men disappeared for a rest break into the shed with Susana's state-of-the-art computer and sound recording equipment. She stood outside the door anxiously peering into the darkness, visions of her backpack being slung, like a bag of potatoes, into some corner tormenting her.

Brunswick, the teenage apprentice of Juan, reassured her, "Everything's okay, everything's okay," as he shouldered her pack under her watchful eye and set off before us. We hiked through tall grasses and dried mud, still holding the impression of the hooves of the cows that have been steadily reducing all the rain forests of the world to grasslands for at least a century now. Looking back at the river, an image of the whole region, converted into a gigantic moor like Devonshire, dotted with sheep and cows and denuded of ancestral forests, came to me.

But then we passed the outer ring of devastation and entered a very different world, hiking through great ringing chambers of vegetation with crowds of squawking parrots passing overhead.

"Watch out for snakes," Brunswick warned me. There had just been a heavy rain, which drives all the creatures that crawl upon the face of the earth out in search of higher ground. I began scanning the trail peripherally for the gleam of serpents.

Then I watched Brunswick walk right over a huge snake lying draped all the way across the path. *"Víbora!!!"* I called out to him.

He whirled around and looked back. His youthful face lit up.

"Do you have a mapacho?" he asked me.

In fact I did. I had bought a neatly tied round bundle of the cigarettes just the day before from a woman who sat in a back alley expertly rolling them by hand, a small wand, papers, and a bag of tobacco at her side. I began looking through my backpack while Brunswick searched through the bushes. When I looked up he was fashioning a prong to trap the snake.

"Is it poisonous?" I asked.

"No. It's a boa of the earth. A mantona. It's just a baby." The snake was about three feet long.

He plunged the prong down right at the base of the boa's neck, holding it pinioned while I lit the mapacho and handed it to him. The snake lashed around as Brunswick blew smoke upon it. Its writhing gradually subsided.

He grinned up at me. "Smoke makes them drunk." He stood up holding the snake tightly at the base of its skull, the body coiled around his arm. "Are you afraid?" he asked.

"No," I said. "I like snakes."

"Then you carry it."

He delicately transferred it to me. I took it and held it firmly at the base of its triangular head, admiring the earth-toned colors and sun-dappled patterns on its body. It wrapped itself tightly around my neck and squeezed.

I gave a comical impression of being strangled to death, my tongue hanging out of my mouth. We laughed and resumed our trek through the jungle.

After an additional half hour's walk, just as the trail began to ascend, we stepped over another obstacle lying across our path. A metal pipe, painted orange, extending in both directions through a corridor slashed into the jungle.

"What's this for?" I asked Brunswick, surprised to see a pipeline running through virgin forest.

"Petróleo," he replied, and shrugged.

Finally we arrived, soaked through with sweat, on a ridge where a pair of benches with little thatched roofs had been constructed, above which a hand-painted sign announced, WELCOME TO MAYANTUYACU.

Susana was already standing looking down into the valley below. Transferring the serpent back to Brunswick, I went to join her.

We had arrived. Looking into the canyon, we beheld a flower-lined path leading down into a terrain dotted with little cabins painted with the patterns of the Shipibo. In their midst were set two huge malocas, right below which, at the very bottom of the slope, a crystal clear river flowed through huge slabs of exposed bedrock. Clouds of vapor rose from the water to the heights of the trees on the opposite bank. So it was true. There was an alchemical river of boiling water running through the heart of Mayantuyacu.

I took Susana's hand. This was the green landscape of my dream, running with resuscitating waters. Susana turned to me and said, "It looks like Shangri-la."

That evening before my first ayahuasca session at Mayantuyacu, I spoke with Juan. I told him about my vision back in the maloca at Takiwasi. He giggled as I described being transformed into an indigena. I asked him if it had been him communicating with me that night.

"Sí," he replied from his hammock, smiling like a boy who had just done a magic trick and was enjoying the effect.

Wondering if we were having a problem in translation, I repeated my question as slowly and clearly as possible. "Yes, it was me," he said, with complete simplicity.

Seeing me stumped he added, "You probably saw me in my aspect as an Indian."

Explaining that he has worked at Takiwasi in the past, he said he checks in there during ceremonies to see what spirits are present and to help out the leaders. The image of the old office buildings with delivery chutes for the mail, whose sudden arrival out of nowhere always bordered on the mysterious for me, came to me. I decided that he had a telepathic chute installed at Takiwasi.

"But Maestro, how did you recognize me?"

"I can sense a mind in search of a new curandero. So I invited you to come."

"Maestro, how is this possible?"

"The spirits of the plants move about the world talking with one another, and if you diet sincerely with them they teach this art. Curanderos use telepathy in healing. *Brujos* do damage to others." Medieval woodcuts of witches riding about on broomsticks intoxicated by datura swirled through my mind.

"For a curandero, plants help sustain life," he said, and went on to speak of Christ *within* the plants. I learned that for Juan, Christianity is realized first in the photosynthesis of sunshine, and that plants—with their roots in the soil and their branches spreading to the sky—act as bridges between worlds. Instead of dwelling in the sky, Christ is literally among us, incarnate in the lilies of the field.

Good god, I thought, *this guy is the real deal.*

In the darkness of the maloca, with the sound of the river of boiling water flowing below, the Maestro sang a boat playing in the whirlpools of the sea, and the whole maloca was transformed and we were on a carefree, delicious ride. He sang very old, mysterious icaros of the ancient peoples of the forest, powerful songs that went from language to language, which to sing transforms one into a member of the indigenous group the song comes from. Within them lay landscapes, maybe pure lands, present in what Debussy called the true essence of music: the silence between the notes. My mind felt it could take wing on the oldest of these icaros, like an eagle, into the sky. I asked the Maestro to sing it over and over again. It was simple like plainchant, pure like the cry of an animal in the early morning, resonant with praise. I noted that whenever Juan concluded an icaro he sang the same little ditty, as if to fix the icaro in us, and then he exhaled vigorously two or three times.

Vapor rising from the river drifted in great luminous columns up over the trees, breaking up into wisps that disappeared into the starry night above. Juan sang to the vapor, and then to the spirit of the river, the little canyon, and its seamless interaction with all levels of creation:

> *Linda quebradita, cómo corren tus aguas,*
> *Tus aguitas ciystalinas, ay ay ay ay ay . . .*
> *Cuando corren tus aguas por encima de la roca*

Ay roquito encantador . . .
Cuando corren tus aguas ya la nube se levanta
Entremedio de las nubes ya se va mi Señor Jesucristo
Ya se van al cielo, ya se van al cielo
Donde brillan las estrellas, con el poder de nuestro Señor Jesucristo.

Beautiful little canyon, how your water flows
Your crystalline waters, ay ay ay ay ay . . .
When your waters flow over the stones
Ay, little stone of enchantment . . .
When your waters flow the cloud arises
Amidst the clouds my Lord Jesus Christ is now ascending
Now they are going to the heavens, now they are going to the
    heavens
Where the stars sparkle with the power of our Lord Jesus Christ.

"The icaros aren't remembered with the mind, are they?" I asked him. "It's the *mariri,* the spirit of the plant we accumulate in our chest that holds the song in our memory. It becomes a plant growing in us, that we can transmit to others so it keeps growing. . . ."

The Maestro nodded his head and sat smiling.

Some days after arriving I poked my head out the door of our cabin and saw the aspect of Juan I had been scrutinizing him for that evening in the restaurant in Pucallpa. Wearing a crown of multicolored feathers, he was crossing the compound barefoot, dressed in an orange and red *cushma*—a full-length woven robe—with an ornamental necklace draped around his neck. In his hand he carried a bow and arrows. No longer the anonymous mestizo on the city streets, here he was in his domain, moving through the natural world as a king. Now I was satisfied. This was the shaman of the deep jungle I had come to study with.

6 The Sacred City

When you see your likeness, you are happy. But when you see your images that came into being before you and neither die nor become visible, how much will you bear!

THE GOSPEL OF THOMAS, SAYING 84

To enter the jungle is to shed the civilized self. It is an encounter recorded as a series of brilliantly plumaged occurrences, pouncing like jaguars and flitting like hummingbirds through memory. A mosaic of images the mind grapples in the aftermath to assemble into a greater coherence.

One of the key pieces in the mosaic was the character of the Maestro and the nature of his art.

Juan began our formal education in *vegetalismo**

---

*The origins of vegetalismo lie in the beginning of the twentieth century, when "mestizos apprenticed themselves with increasing regularity to Indian shamans during the social upheavals of the rubber boom, often after a life-threatening illness from which they had been cured. They in turn had trainees, which resulted in the

143

in the massive central maloca of Mayantuyacu. There we would gather at his consultation table in the back, notebooks, pens, and tape recorders at hand before us, a carving of a mischievous elf occupying the floor beside us.

From our vantage point, the river flowed on its boiling course through a garden of stones and down the canyon below us. Brilliant blue birds called suy suy dove in the vapors and rose to perch on top of a little tree held suspended by a muscular vine over where the river narrowed to a churning chute. From there a continous thrumming arose, like a held chord on some massive violin. Hanging on the rafters of the maloca was a large carved signboard that read, THE CAME RENACO IS SACRED. IT HEALED THE SHAMAN.

There we would sit, waiting expectantly, like students of a favorite professor.

Juan would enter, wearing a clean shirt, smiling and saying, *"Buenos días, chicos!"* We, sitting up straight, would respond, *"Buenos días, Maestro!"* and watch expectantly as he settled into his chair.

Opening the drawer of his desk, he would take out a large sketchbook with his gnarled hands and set it before us.

"Bueno, chicos," he would say. "Today we are going to study the tamamuri tree." Opening the book, he would leaf to the appropriate page and show us a drawing he had made of the tree.

Although the medicine ayahuasca is often spoken of as if it were a single plant, in fact it is a synergistic outcome of the brewing of at least two plants, the woody jungle vine ayahuasca and the delicate DMT-packed leaves of chacruna. Our first day's lesson, therefore, was on chacruna, a beautiful little tree that produces red berries. The spirit of this tree, we learned, is a woman with light skin and hair, dressed in white, who is queen of the forest. Her spirit permeates the forest through the

---

spread of *vegetalismo,* a widespread syncretic mix of herbalism and shamanism in Amazonia."[1] The mestizos also introduced Christ, the Virgin Mary, and, to a lesser extent, the saints, into shamanism, although "the closer to indigenous Amazonian cultures in their training, the less mestizo shamans call upon Catholic sources of power."[2]

circulation of water, which is why she is also a *sirena*—a mermaid.*

As a *doctora,* chacruna paints the visions when her leaves are taken in combination with her mate, the *varón ayahuasca,* the fellow who provides the force and direction, the muscle, for her medicine to flow. He is a spirit that wears a brown hat.

"A brown hat?" I asked the Maestro.

"*Sí,* a brown hat. His skin is also brown, and he wears a white suit."

"Okay." I carefully noted down this description under Juan's watchful eye.

As we continued on through the indigenous pharmacopeia, we began to meet the other doctors of the jungle, those plants with *madres.* While these plants are not blatantly psychoactive like ayahuasca, we learned their spirits and teaching capacity are still the key component to their efficacy as medicine. Juan would describe the preparation of the plant, whether it was grated, pounded or scraped, soaked or boiled, and what part of the plant was used: roots, bark, or leaves. The concoctions were less thick and intensely bitter than ayahusaca, and normal dosages were larger: a small cupful taken three times a day.

Over the days we learned about the pinshacayo plant, whose spirit is the toucan. The pinshacayo has long leaves like the tongue of the bird; its spirit reinforces the body, bones, and blood, and it gives protection. The chullachaqui caspi, a curative and teacher plant, is known as the king of the forest (the statue of the mischievous elf turned out to be him). The tahuarí, who takes the cold out of the body (rheumatism), gives heat, brings good dreams, and teaches how to find other plants that cure. The guacamayo caspi, whose spirit is a parrot of different colors, comes in dreams to teach how to heal. The ajosquiro is a doctor curandero, whose bark must be scraped in the sunshine. The use of it, when dieting, is very strictly monitored; one can die if the diet is not completed properly. Its

---

*Interestingly, chacruna, or *Psychotria viridis,* is a member of the same Rubiaceae family of plants as coffee, that other painter of visions whose shrines, as Dale Pendell has put it, can be found in virtually every office and home across the Western world. For a remarkable discussion on coffee and its imprint upon human consciousness, see his *Pharmakodynamis.*

spirit is a fellow, a doctor with white hair, a white sombrero, and white skin. This plant brings many dreams of spirits and instructions of how to heal, as well as fortifying the body and cleaning the arteries.

"Have no fear of the spirits," Juan added as an afterthought.

And then there is tobacco.

The shamans of the Amazon consider tobacco a food for the spirits, whose smoke the spirits crave like ambrosia. Our own brain sprouts nicotine receptors like leaves when it is fed the molecule and, as with the spirits, the more you give them, the more they want. So central is tobacco to the curandero's art that the Asháninca word for "shaman" is *sheripiári*—one who ingests tobacco.

By this point we had become accustomed to the sight of shamans blowing the smoke of sopladas over their patients. Even the songs of the shamans are hazy with smoke: the word *icaro* is most probably derived from the Quichua* verb *ikaray,* "to blow smoke in order to cure." And we knew that the dark, aromatic leaves of *Nicotiana rustica* we purchased in the markets, rolled up tight in *mazos* like a huge cigar, packed a wallop of nicotine—roughly eighteen times more than the pale and wan *Nicotiana tabacum* consumed in the North, allowing it to be classified as a true psychoactive substance.

In addition to nicotine, "the smoke of tobacco contains nine hundred other constituents. Several of these compounds, including carbon dioxide, myristicin, and nitrous oxide, have known hallucinogenic effects. Harman, an alkaloid similar to the harmine found in *yajé* (ayahuasca), is produced in tobacco smoke, as are many chemical deliriants."[3] It's amusing to consider that the average Joe smoker of a pack of Marlboros is partaking of the same psychoactive effects, albeit on a subliminal level, as the shaman ayahuasqueros of the Amazon.

The wonder of it all, though, is how the curanderos, who are never seen with a Marlboro hanging from their lips, consume massive amounts of the plant—eating, drinking, and snorting it, as well as smoking it (the

*This Quechua dialect is spoken in the northern Peruvian Amazon.

Aztecs even give themselves enemas with it)—and those hale old *tobaque-ros* don't get cancer. No one has studied why this is so, although it may offer the key to understanding what the human species' fascination with tobacco is really all about. But one thing is clear. Among the curanderos, the plant is actually *directed*, utilized as a medicine to cleanse the body and spirit, rather than passively consumed for a high within the addict's spiral of diminishing returns.

Most probably it is not the tobacco that causes cancer, anyway.

Amazonian tobacco is grown without chemical fertilizers or pesticides, and contains none of the ingredients added to cigarettes, such as aluminum oxide, potassium nitrate, ammonium phosphate, polyvinyl acetate, and a hundred or so others, which make up approximately 10 percent of the smokable matter. During combustion, a cigarette emits some 4,000 substances, most of which are toxic. Some of these substances are radioactive in the daily life of an average smoker. According to one study, the average smoker absorbs the equivalent of the radiation dosages from 250 chest X-rays per year.[4]

Tobacco companies appear to corrupt the virtue of tobacco in the same way as the drug cartels corrupt the medicinal coca plant into cocaine.

According to Juan, the spirit of tobacco is *moreno*, a man the same color as the tobacco leaf. He is the director of all plants, which is why the curandero blows its smoke over other plant remedies.

Every part of the tobacco plant is used, from the roots to flowers, which are like little red trumpets. The heated leaf is applied to aches in the joints. *Ampiri*, or tobacco cream, is used to heal wounds, as a disinflammatory, and to treat parasites. A juice of soaked and strained tobacco can be taken as an emetic or laxative or it can be dieted to protect the body, and to ward off bad spirits.

Strange as it may be for us to conceive of plants as allies, perhaps our own priests should consider giving sopladas of tobacco to cleanse penitent sinners after confession. Among the tidbits of information Juan began feeding us, he related the story of a patient who got drawn into the practice of brujería to the point of studying texts on black magic. Juan simply gave him sopladas of tobacco for a couple of weeks, and the man not only recovered his health, but also lost all interest in his occult studies.

The diets sounded severe, and they followed an unvarying regime: no salt, no sugar (including the citric acid in fruit), and no spices. No coffee, tea, alcohol, pork, or beef either. Also, no sexual activity. None. Explanations for this proscription varied, but the essential point seemed to be containing the process of the plants. The human organism is very vulnerable and open in diet, and according to Juan, if a man in diet were to engage in sex with a female partner, she would deplete him energetically. Conversely, a woman would receive all the impurities of her non-dieting male partner. At Takiwasi, this proscription extended explicitly to include masturbation.

Diets have differing degrees of intensity, the strongest involving complete isolation in the jungle. During such periods of withdrawal, which can last as long as months, the dieter eats only plantains, called *inguiri* by locals, some rice, and yucca. Also, Juan always added, you can eat the fish called *boquichico,* which lives in the rivers of the Amazon and feeds only on plants.

"As well, you can cook the root of the tobacco to do diets. One doesn't vomit, but rather one has visions, dreams. The root brings spirits to meet. Especially, the spirit of the tobacco plant itself."

This we were to discover eventually for ourselves.

"Bueno, chicos," Juan would say when he finished his lessons. "Now you draw the plants for yourselves"—and, taking colored pencils and pens out of his desk, he would spread them before us and leave. Feeling just like I was back in elementary school, I searched around for the right shades of brown for bark and green for leaves, red for berries, and yellow for flowers. We sat drawing contentedly, until I noticed something.

"Hey, none of these drawings are botanically accurate. We couldn't identify the leaf of the chacruna with this." The leaves were either small or large in Juan's drawings, done with the fat strokes of felt-tip pens, but there were no details, like the way the spine of the chacruna leaf rises in notches, flaring out a brief distance on either side.

"They're like children's drawings," I added.

"No, they're not," Susana replied impatiently. "Don't you see these are the plants as seen through the eyes of a curandero?"

"Oh," I said, feeling dumb, just like I had in school. I flipped through the pages. Juan had drawn a hundred plants, carefully numbering each one. Some of the trees had faces peering out of the trunks, just as in Pablo Amaringo's visionary landscapes.

But I remained unconvinced, until Juan delivered a skillful blow to my skepticism.

The Cocina para Medicinas was located down the hill from the maloca, over a bridge that crossed a boiling little stream that fed into the river below. Past luxuriant growths of basil and flowers, it lay at a spot where the river forked and flowed off in directions only the low-flying carrion eaters could follow.

The "Medicine Kitchen" was a typical jungle structure: packed-earth floor, posts of tree trunks still swathed in their bark, and a roof of woven palm fronds. Squarish boulders were set, clean and smooth as molars, into the earth around the fire pit, where huge logs were fed into the flames that licked the hot, vapor-laden air throughout the day. Gigantic pots and ladles sat on shelves on the far end of the structure. Brunswick, in the way of all teenagers, had declared it his domain by writing his name down on one of the posts.

It was a good place to hang out. Sitting with Brunswick, Susana and I took up another part of our education: the harvesting and preparation of the medicines we had come to study. While clumsily wielding machetes to scrape bark or split vine, we smoked mapachos and got to know one another. Brunswick spoke with a fluted accent that I initially found difficult to comprehend, and which had the effect of reducing our conversation to the groping minimum. By then, however, I was learning that the people of the jungle don't measure successful communication by self-disclosure—it's what gets done that counts.

That morning Juan had been circling us with an ax in his hand for some time, and finally he came in and sat with us. He wore a green cap molded over his indigenous features, reminding me of Yoda, especially in the way his facial muscles fanned out laterally across his face whenever he smiled.

"So you're learning how to prepare the plants," he said approvingly, leaning his ax against a log. "Very good. It's important to know the plants, how to harvest them and prepare them."

Sitting on one of the stumps that served as a bench, he took out a mapacho, lit it, and blew little puffs of smoke on both sides of his body before settling back to talk. He made polite queries about how we were accustoming ourselves to the jungle, and after a while we began talking about the doctors of the plants we were preparing, and how they teach.

Describing ayahuasca as the university of the forest, Juan told us that through the archives preserved in the leaf of the plant one can major, for example, in art. He had seen, playing before him in vast panoramas, the art of the ancient Egyptians, of the Incans, Chinese, and Mayans. Within the plants there are no limits to the living worlds that can be read, he said, once one learns how to direct the mind.

This reminded me of a certain modern theory in physics, which, to account for the nonspatial and nontemporal features of quantum reality, postulates that the universe is a hologram, in which each part contains a faithful image of the whole. Each cell, each molecule, each electron, "enfolding" the entire cosmos within it, contains "archives" of all events— past, present, and future. And since the brain is also an integral part of that hologram, theoretically there is no obstacle preventing us from "reading" those archives once we get over our habit of lurking exclusively within the province of our gray matter.

Then Juan pulled the rug out from beneath us.

"You two are very educated people," he said. "I would like to ask you a question."

"Go ahead, Maestro," I said, expecting an obtuse query about Western science or philosophy.

"God is the creator of the universe, yes? And it's said that everything we see and experience has its source in him. Bueno, is there something that God doesn't know?"

A silence followed.

Juan wore a poker face. Was he asking this question with the humility he was displaying? Or was he setting a trap for our "educated" minds to fall into?

Listening to Susana's description of how Vedanta philosophy would answer that question, he displayed no indication that he took his question in any way but seriously.

Is there something that God doesn't know? I asked myself. The question smacked of heresy, something out of the old beliefs of the Gnostics.

But Juan didn't seem out to undermine Yahweh, at least not deliberately. His question was far deeper than the metaphysical, I decided. I felt that existential vertigo one gets when confronting the koans of the Zen masters of old, who posed questions such as, "What is the sound of a single hand?" or "Say something without moving your lips and tongue." A direct pointing to the nature of mind, the old texts say, cutting off the mind road.

"Maestro," I said, "there is an ancient question in the Buddhist tradition: When the entire universe is consumed by fire at the end of the world age, is Buddha nature consumed as well? Your question strikes me as similar."

Juan nodded. Then he said, "Since I don't know anything that is outside of myself, how can God know what is outside of himself?"

Watching him rise and take his ax in his hand, it occurred to me we had just received a sly lesson outside classroom ethnobotany—this one in the style of the Asháninca, who transmit their knowledge orally, through encounters, independent of the written word.

Some days later, a priest, musicians, and several scores of celebrants trundled down the river and through the jungle to help Mayantuyacu celebrate the *velada* to El Señor de los Milagros on October 18, along with the rest of Peru, with all-night dancing and prayer.

A couple years previous, Juan had wandered lost in the jungle for five days, causing a distraught Sandra to vow to throw the traditional celebration for the saint at Mayantuyacu if Juan emerged safely. So in the central maloca, lit up with candles and caressed by clouds of vapor rising from the river below, we danced in rows to the sound of the fife and drum. An old Spanish processional dance, one where we held hands and beat out the rhythm with our feet as we circled the maloca, pausing to dance in place before the altars that had been erected to venerate the saints enshrined there: El Señor de los Milagros and San Martín de Porres.

A fat, expansive priest offered Mass, and we sang a hymn called "The People of the Forest Praise You, Lord." During the dancing, I noticed this all-night festival was also an opportunity for the young people, separated by wide distances in the jungle, to court and flirt. At least one baby was conceived in honor of the saint that evening.

Beating out the medieval rhythm in place before the mulatto figure of San Martín felt particularly appropriate at Mayantuyacu. As an herbalist and founder of the first hospital in Lima, he is venerated by curanderos for introducing the indigenous knowledge of plants to the new European culture. Depictions of San Martín show him dressed in the black robe of a Dominican and holding a broom in his right hand. In a manner reminiscent of St. Francis, a dog, a cat, and a rat are seen feeding peacefully together from a single dish before him.

Unable to keep my eyes open after hours of dancing, I descended to the river and lay on the smooth slabs of exposed bedrock, contemplating the glowing maloca and the stars above. I went to sleep that night with the sound of the drum beating in the distance like a comforting rain on the roof.

In the totality of creatures that inhabit the jungle, humans are but a minor presence.

There were cloudless nights in the valley where the stars were shining, and the sky was filled with silent, spectral fire. *Relámpago seco*. Dry lightning: sudden expanding balls of light coming down from the hills, eerily silent, exploding so close to the earth they seemed to emerge from within it. The people at Mayantuyacu said the spirits were congregating in the hills.

The biting insects, maddened by the blazing white lights, would burn our skins and drive us beneath our mosquito nets for shelter. It was the rainy season, and after the deluges the insects would come seeking shelter, ravenous for food and blood. Huge spiders with long, bony legs and beady eyes appeared on our walls, so persistent that if I had managed to only wound them with my machete, they would later reappear in the same spot, missing a leg or two. Occasional tarantulas, big and hairy as spiny cactuses, would arise between the floorboards of our cottage and stalk through. Cockroaches scuttled everywhere, licking the sheen of protein off anything left unwashed.

Ants ferreted out openings in our containers of evaporated milk and nibbled at the pages of older books. Giant winged beetles wandered around like cows. Gangs of diabolical mosquitoes buzzed in the ears, passing unimpeded through the open slats in our walls, miraculously materializing in our mosquito nets while we slept. Wasps built nests overnight in our eaves and dead husks of curled-up spiders fell from the ceiling like dust. And then there were the truly exotic, otherworldly, long-limbed jewel-studded insects we would encounter in the jungle, displaying unimaginable forms and adaptations that sent chills up the spine, or took our breath away.

Insect repellent only halted their assaults briefly. Our bodies became pebbled with bites, our feet and arms deformed, and eventually the situation was so surreal that an animal-like indifference began to envelop us. We were, however, compelled to make peace with them. If we must share our planet with this parallel form of life—armor-plated, beady-eyed, calculating, and ravenous—we decided that we had better start appealing to their intelligence.

Susana struck the first deal with the spiders. "Okay," she announced as if she were on the public address system. "You spiders are good and we like you, but you are not permitted inside the house or in the outhouse! We don't want to kill you, but we will if you come inside!" That seemed to do the trick, and I no longer had to precede Susana into the outhouse with my machete. Then, one week our hands and feet began to resume their normal smooth contour. We were being bitten just the same, but our systems had adapted.

But when the rats began crawling beneath our door, climbing our walls and waking us up in the night fighting in the thatched roof, Susana had had enough. It was time to strike back.

Our stealth weapon traveled the final stretch to Mayantuyacu curled up in a little ball in Susana's handbag. When we delicately removed the black-and-white-striped kitten from the safety of the pouch to face the new world in the jungle, she kept her eyes shut tight. Carefully laying her in a cardboard box, we covered the top with a thin towel to keep the mosquitoes from molesting her. Soaking cat food in milk, I mashed it up and we fed her by dipping the end of a rag in it and giving it to her to suck. Soon she made her first trembling forays across the floor. We named her Tigrilla, after one of the midsized wildcats of Peru.

I made her a litter box and we took shifts feeding her, but my paternal instinct was not aroused. Susana, on the verge of leaving for Lima for a week-long conference, buttonholed me and stated flatly, "You don't seem to realize we have a cat in our care here. This creature is totally dependent on us."

"What's there to realize? It's a cat and I'm going to take care of it. What are you worried about?" I asked, slightly annoyed.

Susana left downriver on the Pachitea and I walked home, opened the door to the cabin, and flopped on the bed. Looking around the room, I contemplated my week of bachelorhood.

Tigrilla never mewed, and she never came seeking affection out of need. I fed her and kept an eye on her water bowl. She instantly worked out the litter box and already knew how to keep herself clean. I petted her as a matter of course—the friendly giant. She made it out onto the deck on her quivering new legs and sat beside me staring at the big world as I smoked. All the hens foraging around the kitchen cocked their heads and took careful note of her. Thus we passed a couple of days in peaceful cohabitation.

Then came the evening of work with ayahuasca, and in the darkness of the early morning when I returned, lighting the lamp and moving about the room, Tigrilla stirred and clambered out of her box where I had left her to sleep. She was hungry, and I fed her as the high-voltage currents of the plant still coursed through my body. Then we played. Not the conventional dangle-the-fuzzy-object-for-the-cat-to-bat-with-its-little-paw, but a communication of two animals immersed in the jungle. I was struck with wonder at the emerging intelligence of the little cat. How quick to apprehend—how perfectly attuned with her environment she was. I admired her. It was like watching a butterfly bursting forth with wings.

Tigrilla and I decided we liked each other, and we began to hang out more. Outside of wild ayahuasca visions of jaguars, I had not been close to a cat since my childhood, and it was refreshing.

In my subsequent session with ayahausca, I began having visions of Tigrilla: of her accompanying me with delicate steps, of her intelligence softening the hard edges of my experience with gentler, more playful approaches. After the session was over, I walked back up to the cabin and opened the door, my headlamp blazing with stellar light into the darkness. There she was, sitting in the middle of the hardwood floor.

"Oh, you are a good one," I told her.

Soon whenever I sat down to meditate she would come and clamber over my knees to curl up in the cup of my hands.

We now had a cat. But Tigrilla was turning out to be more than a mere pet—she was showing signs of taking on the traditional role of a familiar, an animal that serves as a bridge and mediator between worlds. Sometime later, lying beneath my mosquito net after an ayahuasca session, the face of a Shipiba witch suddenly swam into view. I saw how she had been feeding off my sensory field since that vulnerable day with don Martín in San Francisco. In an instinctive response that I suspect belongs to our genetic inheritance, just like convulsive vomiting or the fight-or-flight instinct, I treated her as an invasive entity and cast her out.

As I lay there contemplating the night of the jungle outside, the teeming witches' brew of evolution, I turned to stroke Tigrilla.

I was startled to see the structure of her face transformed: a divine being of infinite love and compassion was looking back at me through her eyes.

By the time Susana returned, Tigrilla was on dry food and aggressively mastering her environment and I was in the full bloom of proud parenthood.

Susana, however, was in crisis. We had been in the Peruvian Amazon for months, and however rich the learning experience may have been, she still had no bona fide participants for her study. Takiwasi, with its resident population and regimen of treatment, had been ideal, but the center had lost their Cocama ayahuasquero and hadn't moved to contract another mestizo curandero.

Then there were the other obstacles that had arisen: the magical and primitive thinking of the trade (MONEY, LOVE AND LUCK written over a poker hand with four aces painted on a curandera's storefront); the suspicion of foreigners (narrowed eyes regarding us coolly from hammocks hung in dim interiors); the lack of a conceptual framework to incorporate a concept such as "profound healing" (candles flickering before portraits of saints in gold-gilded frames, flecks of mold accumulating behind the glass); a lack of structure and continuity (ayahuasca tourists looking disoriented in front of the curandero's wide-screen television); and finally there was all the witchcraft and hexing that was going on.

Susana had led us through it all to Mayantuyacu, and now that conditions seemed ideal there were no patients in residence and no word of any coming.

Besides us, there were only two other residents at the center. One was a tall, blond French woman who was withdrawn into the strictest diet, living in a maloca on top of a hill and speaking to no one but the Maestro and those who brought her the plants. The other resident, a young American athlete with a taste for esoteric theories, had come as a student, not as a patient. He practiced icaros and dieted and studied nutrition and the energies of the body. Neither one appeared to be possibilities for Susana's study.

Even as we carefully recorded and documented our ayahausca sessions, Susana's sense of desperation had mounted.

"Yes, this place is wonderful. But even if it is Shangri-la, it's not going to be of use to my study if there are no participants. We can't just sit around and hope for the best," she said, replying to my objection that we had just arrived at the ideal place.

"We, or at least I, are going to have to leave if Juan doesn't start receiving patients."

"Well, let's talk with him."

Juan listened attentively to Susana's concerns, and then he asked one question: "By what date do you need to complete your study?"

"January 21," she answered.

"Let me see what I can do," he told her.

A few days later he called us to his consulting table in the central maloca, where he and Sandra sat awaiting us with a formal air. "You will have your healing experiences by January 21," he told Susana.

She and I glanced at each other. From his tone, it was obvious that he had consulted the spirits, and there was no better assurance to receive from a curandero. We accepted his word without reservation.

I breathed a deep sigh of relief. I had no desire to leave this valley.

Brunswick came and sat down across from me one morning as I addressed myself to a plate of rice and lentils without salt. He had a tranquil but expressive face, and when he regarded things with his deep brown eyes, his gaze was completely unsocialized. He looked until he saw what he needed to see, and beyond that he couldn't be bothered. In a similar way, his movements showed an easy spontaneity rarely encountered among civilized folk with hardened personas.

That morning Brunswick's head was freshly shaved. He dug into a plate of roast yucca while he narrated a dream he had had the night before. I was coming to understand his singsong accent better and followed with interest his account of "interviewing" the spirits.

Brunswick had come to Mayantuyacu fresh out of the military with a serious alcohol dependency. After curing himself, he stayed on as Juan's apprentice. We had not realized his status until one evening, when, at the nether end of a ceremony, a sound arose in the darkness of the maloca that seemed to come from some subterranean region of grinding agony.

It was Brunswick singing.

Before long I saw out of the corner of my eye the white figure of Susana arising and leaving the maloca, but I stuck it out, telling myself I was seeing a new aspect of Amazonian culture and should stay to support the debut of a young curandero. But as he enumerated the plants, calling each one to him and asking it to heal him, his voice did not improve and finally when the moaning and dragging of chains showed no sign of subsiding, I discreetly exited as well.

We had since learned that Brunswick was a remarkably sensitive apprentice curandero, and that his soul was not in torment. He simply didn't know how to carry a tune. That morning he invited me to go into the jungle to harvest came renaco, a plant with healing properties for bone and muscle that I was to start drinking for an injury I had in my lower back.

The plant came renaco is the one praised as sacred on the carved signboard prominently hung in the maloca, a tribute that came to be there because of a pivotal event that occurred during the early days of Mayantuyacu.

Out gathering plants one late afternoon, Juan made the fateful decision to collect just one more chiric sanango growing at the bottom of a slope. As he took his final step to reach the plant, his foot caught the trip-wire of a trap and a shotgun went off point-blank into his legs, shattering one of his tibia. With his flesh ragged and rapidly losing blood, Juan was carried out in a hammock and taken downriver to get a car to the clinic.

Upon arrival, the doctors said he probably only had a couple of hours to live. They replaced his shattered bone with steel plates and gave him a blood transfusion, but it was because of the plants he had dieted for so many years, plants whose blood was already in his body, Juan says, that he did not die.

After only a week, Juan returned to Mayantuyacu, where he soon set aside his antibiotics and began dieting with came renaco, tamamuri, and other plants. He dreamt of their spirits coming and removing his cast, massaging, and bathing his wounded legs. After eight months, Juan was limping around with a cane. Then one night he dreamt the spirits told him to drop the cane and run three times up and down a hill. He did so, and when he awoke he never used a support again. By the time I met him, he didn't even have a limp and was rambling through the jungle.

It was a fine day for a walk to visit the tree, so after eating we set off, Brunswick swinging a machete at his side.

As we rose out of the valley, Brunswick took a path I had not yet followed, and we soon entered the presence of gigantic, buttressed trees with vines dangling like serpents from their canopies. Palm fronds twice my height reached to the sun filtering through the emerald vault above, supported by massive trees arrayed like the pillars of Gothic architecture. I was filled with the kind of happiness I experience strolling in a medieval cathedral.

But then I thought of Juan's words to us, that one must truly love nature and the plants to do a shaman's work. I realized that I loved nature, but it was more the noble nature of Ansel Adams, Emerson, and Thoreau. To love plants in the shamanic world is to love their spirits, to trust them and fully enter into their realm. We civilized types adore our coffee, tea, tobacco, and wine—all gifts from plants—but could I love the came renaco that I was about to drink as medicine?

Brunswick halted before me, running his hand affectionately down the trunk of a small tree with stilt roots. "This is the Chulla Chaqui Caspi," he said, "the king of the jungle. He brings the animals and teaches how to walk in the forest."

The bark of the plant was mottled green and gray, and I didn't quite know how he had picked it out from the other surrounding trees.

"When you diet with him he teaches you about the plants in the jungle, but he can be dangerous too. He likes to trick people and lead them astray in the woods."

"Okay," I said, feeling overwhelmed with information in the midst of so much anonymous green.

"He likes to kick the trees with his clubfoot before it rains, and you can hear the sound ringing through the forest," Brunswick added, then nodded his head, satisfied. We set off again.

Arriving at the summit of a steep hill, we halted and faced a tall tree half swallowed up by a vine. Then I understood the origin of the truly massive, Gothic-looking specimens we had passed on the way. What had begun as a single dangling string reaching down from an epiphytic plant in the canopy heights had taken root, and then swollen into a muscular giant that would finally elbow its host out of existence.

"The tree is a came renaco?" I asked.

"No," said Brunswick. "The vine is," he said, and he patted it affectionately. Ahh. So I was to drink the vine. . . .

Lighting a mapacho, Brunswick carefully blew smoke on the plant. Then we followed its tentacles to the base of the hill and dug out an area where it entered a little stream. Brunswick blew more smoke on it and cut out a section. White sap began to pour from its severed ends.

Immediately dropping down on his hands and knees, Brunswick began to drink it, looking, for all the world, like a child catching milk squirting from a cow's udder. I cupped some in the palm of my hand and lapped it up. It had the consistency of rubber and a neutral taste.

Clambering back up the hill, we sat and smoked mapachos. Then leaving the butt ends burning upright at the base of the plant as an offering, we returned home to our respective tasks: Brunswick to prepare the medicine and I to find out if I could love the spirit of a strangler jungle vine.

Susana, meanwhile, had begun, at the recommendation of the Maestro, dieting chacruna, the queen of the forest who paints the visions in ayahuasca. I often found her sitting on the steps of our cabin smoking her pipe, absorbed in knitting tobacco bags and necklaces. She reported her senses were becoming more delicate, colors were brighter and the world subtler, as if the feminine receptivity of the plant were working in her. During our sessions, she found herself traveling more through the jungle in her visions, following the waterways of the plant.

I soon found myself descending to the shores of the river and stroking the muscular limbs of the came renaco vine. Wholly absorbed in its tenacious strength, feeling its power running through my body, I began crooning to it like a lover.

The episode of the toucans began with a morning excursion. Ascending out of the valley with our friend Mireya, a Mexican psychotherapist who, like Susana, was also a holotropic breathworker, we came upon Tigrilla sunning herself on the deck of our cabin. She had been filling out and was no longer wobbling around beneath a huge head. She raced instead and clambered the walls and rafters. One morning I heard a rustling in the thatched roof, and I was dismayed to see her head poking through. She was developing special walks too. Our favorite was the cakewalk, where she would angle her body sideways and dance toward us across the narrow deck that ran around our cabin. It was a special prance, designed specifically to let us know that she knew she was the apple of our eye.

We continued relating to her in both worlds. As she clambered the rafters she clambered our ayahuasca visions, the third member of our unity, winding her purring, tenaciously clawing self through our confrontations with our own unconscious and the inhabitants of the landscape of spirit.*

Returning at the end of a session, we would hear her calling us as we

---

*Even as I lie in a hammock writing this, many moon's distance from these events, a beautiful black and red hummingbird, the messenger spirit in Amazonian cosmology, has come, flitting straight through the center of Mayantuyacu's maloca—a sight never seen in all my time here.

approached the cabin, and opening the door it was as if we were back from long, perilous journeys and the world was whole again.

Nights Susana and I would rest together in one of our beds, our heads touching, feeling our consciousness merging in the same mysterious sea, our Tigrilla nestled between us, dreaming her own cat dreams. One night, we beheld her on her back, her paws and legs in the air, an expression of beatific feline contentment on her face.

Susana caressed her with a little finger beneath her chin. "You were born under a lucky star," she told her.

That particular morning, as we prepared to hike out of the valley, Susana stopped and fixed her eyes on the three-month-old Tigrilla.

"C'mon Tigrilla, let's go for a walk."

Tigrilla looked confused, and Susana half turned, and, motioning uphill, said again, "C'mon, little one, let's go."

Tigrilla continued to stare, as Mireya and I watched.

"C'mon."

I was about to open my mouth and say, "Cats don't walk with people like dogs do, Susana," when, with a little bound, Tigrilla was off the deck and accompanying us up the hill. Mireya and I looked at each other, stunned. And if we thought she was going to drop off, we were wrong too. Once committed, the cat stuck, bounding along beside us through what for her were tall grasses and steep ledges out of the valley. When we reached the river, she needed some coaxing, but soon she was leaping over the boulders, skirting steaming cauldrons of boiling water, letting herself be carried over jumbles of stone, and coasting through the smooth, dry channels cut in the bedrock by generations of torrents flowing from above.

We visited Carlos, who was dieting far back in the jungle in a tiny maloca called a *tambo* in Quechua—"resting place." He was located at a confluence of streams, eating a very simple fare of roast green bananas and rice, lying beneath his mosquito net and watching the days flow by. Carlos had been deeply affected by an icaro in a recent session and was now a participant in Susana's study. So while she stayed to chat with him and Mireya rested, I climbed the next ridge, Tigrilla bounding up alongside me. She was beginning to pant and stumble, so I picked her up and carried her.

Reaching the ridge, I set her down and we entered more deeply into the trees. Suddenly, there came a ruckus from the canopy—a squawking and a loud flapping of wings. Frozen in place, Tigrilla and I watched as a troop of toucans came crashing through, their beaks impossibly huge and brilliant, their bodies black with splashes of red and yellow. One flew almost directly across the path in front of me, a slow-motion, meteoric rainbow.

We remained stock-still as their raucous progress receded into the distance. I had never seen a toucan before, except on the cover of a cereal box. I felt graced.

A couple of nights later, after a session, the Maestro, Brunswick, Susana, and I were lying around on a pile of mattresses when the Maestro said to Brunswick, "Go get that gift I wanted to give Robert." Brunswick nodded his head and left the maloca.

When he returned, he handed an object wrapped in cloth to the Maestro. As Susana and I watched expectantly, the Maestro unrolled it and took out a toucan's beak, skull firmly attached. He handed it to me, and I turned it over in my hands in wonder.

"It's a totem! Maestro, we will always have this on the altar when we do ceremonies," Susana said.

"Yes, and when I write I will have it on my desk," I chimed in.

The Maestro used the word *pinsha* to refer to the toucan, and he told us how, as a young curandero, he would sing huarmi icaros when he was in love with a woman. If the woman heard the call of the pinsha at sunset and started to cry for no reason, Juan knew his icaro had taken effect.

Holding that toucan's beak, swept up in the romance of it all, I suddenly wanted to be a full-fledged curandero.

"Where does the beak come from?" I asked him.

"I was walking through the jungle one day with my rifle and a flock of pinshas came through. I wanted to see if I still shot as well as I had in my youth."

I knew this meant something beyond mere marksmanship. Lately, Juan had taken to saying to me, *"Dispara bien!"* "Shoot straight!" I was dieting with the plant chuchuwasi, which, the Maestro had explained to me, teaches a shaman how to shoot, and when he had sufficient power, to hit the medicinal target.

I held up the beak in my hands and bowed to him over it. He reached out and took it, and then he placed his fingers at its delicately hooked mouth.

"If you have any trouble passing through customs, make it call: *'Tío Juan! Tío Juan!'"* he said, animating the beak and drawing out the words "Uncle John" to sound like a toucan's call.

We burst into laughter. The image of the beak calling the Maestro was forever engraved upon my gift.

Dieting is one of the great arts of the jungle, we were learning from the Maestro, particularly at the conclusion of a ceremony with ayahuasca, when Juan would grow expansive and address the small circle gathered around him, holding us, rapt with his jungle lore.

The shamans of old were hardy fellows and, by following strict diets with the plants, had achieved such feats as rejuvenating themselves or rendering themselves invisible at will. They had also learned how to become jaguars, he told me one evening while I was still *mareado,* his face looking wizened and ancient below his Yoda cap in the dancing colors of the darkness.

"Jaguars?" I asked, with the rising excitement of a little kid being told stories around a campfire. A tide of hilarity arose in me as the cat stirred inside.

"Yes, they could transform into a cat and go visit people."

In my *mareación,* I half-expected a cat to burst out of him right there, like the half cat and half human theriomorphic deities sculpted by the ancient peoples of the jaguar in Mexico.

Other nights, he told us about seeking "interviews" with spirits and how essential this was to a shaman's development. He then related this tale from his own days of study:

Ever since I was very young, I wanted to be a curandero. My father was a curandero, and my mother interpreted the messages of animals and birds. I always watched how my father harvested and prepared plants. I also took food to him when he dieted in the forest, where he would live for a week, two weeks, or even a month in a little hut, drinking preparations from different plants, and eating only green bananas and yucca.

I never had a chance to take ayahuasca with him, but I watched how he prepared it and healed his patients. One day he went to work for a man he was healing and he forgot his tobacco bag. When my mother saw it sitting out with his pipe she knew he was unprotected and something bad was going to happen. I ran to take him his tobacco, but I was too late. The spell he was trying to remove was too powerful—from a shaman of the opposition—and a falling tree killed him that day.

I began to study at age ten with the maestro Abel Dávila. I was afraid he would not accept me because of my youth, so I was very happy when he did.

After three years I began to cure children. Sometimes children encounter bad spirits, spirits of the dead, and it always spooks them badly. I would also gather my friends, saying, "Hey, c'mon guys, let's drink ayahuasca together!" and I would sing the songs I had learned from my master for them. By the time I was nineteen I was curing adults with serious diseases, and I began to travel through Peru, spending time in the native communities, learning their medicines, how they prepared them, how they healed people, and above all how they communed with the plant.

I was with the Shipibo, as well as the Cashibo that come from the river Waitea, with the Yaminawas in the Alto Ucayali, with the Matsigenka on the Río Tambo, and with the curanderos in the folds of the Madre de Dios Mountains. I went from community to community, sometimes staying six months, sometimes a year. My greatest desire was, and still is, to know and know more.

I also liked, and still like, to find where the strongest spirits are so I can learn from them. It's an idea I've had ever since I was very young.

Spirits like to live in the mountains and in the most silent places in the jungle. They don't like noise. So I would go to these places to learn from them and receive teaching, but the communication is by means of the plants, the diets—when one drinks ayahuasca, the spirits come to talk. It can happen at any moment. There's no set hour. They come in dreams, visions, during ceremonies, or while you are hanging in a hammock smoking tobacco. In those places the patient can feel the energy arriving through the plants. That's what I discovered long, long ago, and now I continue studying, because the study of plants never ends.

In the '80s I had a friend who knew a place where there were many spirits. I sought him for three years, and I finally found him in a little town called Santa Rosa de Masisea. I arrived with my friend, Geraldo González, who, like me, was the son of a curandero. We roped my friend into doing an ayahuasca session with us, and afterward I told him I wanted to talk with the spirits in the place he knew. He agreed. For three days we gathered everything we needed for the journey, and then we left in the morning in a canoe.

Going upriver, the way was dense with renacales, stretches of massive trees whose roots form nearly impassible barriers. It was slow going, and entirely by canoe because in the winter there is almost no bare land, only little ridges above the waterline. Our guide climbed high trees in order to orient us toward the site where the spirits gathered. It was a marvelous journey for me.

When we arrived at the place it was a lagoon, one that formed every twenty-four hours when a canyon opened in the mountain. Other times there was no lake. There was nothing. These mountains open and close, covering their tracks entirely, and they move around as well. When they close, there is nothing. And they can make themselves as visible or invisible as they want. Nothing passes there, not a canoe, not a single boat.

When we arrived at the site the water was very dark. One could see one's face in it. We were a little frightened, and we continued on a little and entered some fifty meters to find a piece of dry land. We arrived and I said, "Well, let's make some noise. Let's fell a tree to find out what kind of creatures are here." I always like to exercise some caution, no? So we cut down a tree and there was nothing. Complete silence. It was already late afternoon, so we stopped there for the night. We constructed a tambito to stay beneath.

I said to them, "Good, now we're going to see. Today we will take ayahuasca in order to see the spirits," and four of them said to me, "Yes, let's drink," but two others were afraid and said no, one of them being our guide! He hadn't quite realized what he was getting himself into. . . .

Anyway, drink we did and around eight o'clock, the mountain began to come alive. Many animals came, moving all around. Now we had to stay put, but we weren't afraid, at least not at first.

Then my friend Geraldo called out to me, "They're coming to carry us away! They're coming to eat us!" We prepared the gun and lamp and gathered together, but there was nothing.

"Maestro," he said to me, "it's the spirits trying to confuse us. We have to smoke." So we lit a few mapachos and smoked. It wasn't five minutes later that the spirit boat came. First we heard its sound, a low humming of an engine, and then the boat came from the water, from the depths of the lake. You see, the lake is shaped like a half-moon, and the ship travels from one side of the lake to the other. It's a very large ship, made of metal, and you can see the doctors and doctoras, the doctoras wearing blue blouses with white skirts.

They're all specialists in everything that concerns medicine. They come to help this world and do their work with those who require it. Our ship is white. Everything associated with the science of medicine is all white, and very well lit. It's just like I sing in the icaro of the whirlpools. But there are others that are dark, no? Those ships are from the negative side, the opposition. With them you can hear their movement, but you can never see them.

I wanted to encounter the ancient doctors and curanderos that exist on the other side as spirits in order to converse with them, to find out how they saw me as a curandero and if they would accept me. They knew everything about my behavior, my way of thinking, because I am someone who has no other agenda. I simply want to learn. If they had not accepted me, I wouldn't have returned to this life. But I went to them healthy and peaceful, and I returned healthy and peaceful.

When we saw them we began to drink ayahuasca and we entered into conversation with them. It was a strong mareación and a marvelous interview we had, getting to know the curanderos of the past.

There was a señor there named Juan José Inuma. He was a shaman from long ago and knew how to dive into the waters. He would say to the children, "Okay, kids, today I'm going to make a movie!" So they would follow him down to the river and he would go into the water. He would make a big whirlpool and go in and come out with a chair in his hand. All the kids would laugh, because he was making such a great movie. Then he would go under again and would change into a dolphin. He was no longer Juan José Inuma, but a dolphin instead. He could transform himself into many different forms, because he had dieted with many plants and arrived at this point.

I was also able to meet Fiscarreal Carraza, another Ashaninca, and Demetrio González too—everyone who had done very strict diets and good work with the plants and had arrived at transformation. And there were doctors from other countries also, from Japan, the United States, Europe, and India. . . .

And there were women in the boat weaving. They were sirenas, doctoras. From the bottom of the waters came the culture of knitting and weaving. The sirenas know all the arts, and they taught them to the Incas. For that reason they say that from the waters of lake Titicaca emerged a couple: Manco Capac and Mama Ocllo. Mama Ocllo was the woman who taught the women on the earth how to weave. This is true, because one can see how the mermaids sew. It's a very mysterious thing. They came from the bottom of the waters to teach their culture to the people of the land and they are all dedicated to healing.

Well, more than anything else I wanted to interview them and ask them if, in the future, I could be in contact with them. Would they come and protect us and help us when I called them? This was my request. It was the most primordial interview I ever had, and I want to transmit it to you now.

Preparing to leave in the morning, we did a turn around the lake in the canoes to say good-bye. We smoked mapachos, and we gave a soplada to the lake. Suddenly it began to rain lightly, the kind of rain that comes with rainbows. So we knew that the Sumiruna that lived in the lake had power and was making the rain fall. Going all around, we were left with very strong impressions. The place was very powerful.

Then when we were in the middle of the lake, we saw the yacumama, the anaconda of the water, rise.

The yacumama is an animal that has power. They live mainly in the water, climbing the renacales. But they also transform and go about everywhere, in this place and that place . . . They are spirits at the same time as they are animals, like the doctor, mermaid, princess . . . Those are three names, but in the end they mean the same: the Sumiruna. The most accomplished doctor of the water, the yacumama, the boa.

We were a bit frightened it had come to eat us. There was no escape. We were in two canoes, and our guide, in order that it would eat all of us together, rowed his canoe over to join us! The yacumama began winding around our canoe, band by band.

Then the pilot of our boat said, "No, we have to smoke. Nothing is going to happen. It's one of us, a friend."

Then he added, "And if it's not a friend, well, we're going to get eaten right in the middle of this lake." So we smoked and continued moving forward, and the yacumama released us and slowly settled back into the water. Nothing happened. The place was very tranquil.

Returning to our campsite, we gathered up our things, and said, "Okay, spirits, we're going now! Now we have met and done our interviews. We hope there will be an opportunity to return."

So these are the people who give their knowledge to this world, to the land where we belong. This is why we have to learn about the plants

of the water, the plants of the land and of space, and how we enter it in
order to receive information from them.

It seemed Susana and I were breaking up in wordless recrimination. The
loner in me had been resurfacing, with his hard edges and gaping lacunae
in relationship skills. Caught in my cycle of deepening isolation, I began
planning a trip to the heights of Machu Picchu, to feel stone in the mountains again, cold and wide skies to lift my spirits, dragging me down like an
anchor weighted with sadness. I would begin my roaming again. Perhaps
that's all I would ever be: a wanderer, or a pilgrim if I wanted to ennoble my
status. Or a vagabond, perhaps, as those who don't like me call me.

I posed the question to ayahuasca before the session began: Do I have
the capacity to form a family with the kind of history I carry?

I drank from the bitter little vessel carved of *palo de sangre* and crawled
beneath my mosquito net. I sat up a very long time but, overwhelmed with
drowsiness, I lay down and drifted off. The Maestro began to sing, and
Susana burst into tears beside me. I listened to her sobs merging with the
sound of the water below. Finally, I was aware that Brunswick was next to
me. It was time for me to go forward to receive a soplada from the Maestro. Afterward, I drank again.

"*Vas a gritar,*" he said. "You're going to scream."

"*Está bien conmigo,*" I answered. "It's okay with me."

I went and sat in a reclining chair to stay awake. Then I noticed an
exquisite light shining through the distant trees.

Oh, the moon is rising, I thought. It arose in splendor, cresting the
trees, half full, and began mounting the sky.

Suddenly the Maestro's voice broke out:

Qué lindo sale la luna	How beautifully comes forth the moon
Alumbrando todo el mundo	Illuminating all the world
Por eso Dios nos ha puesto	For that reason God has put us here

Alumbrando todo el mundo	Illuminating all the world
Estrellita Icunanta	Little star Icunanta
Que alumbra mi camino	That lights my way
Qué linda virgencitaini	Such a beautiful little virgin
Sentadita ayrunacitai	Seated ayrunacitai
En su altarcito ayruna	In her little altar ayruna
Virgencita Icunanta	Little virgin Icunanta

Content, I went and lay beneath my mosquito net again and went back to sleep. I awoke and the session was ending. Going up to the Maestro, I told him there had been no mareación that evening.

"You drank a lot," he said.

"*Sí.*"

He sang the icaro of the ayahuasca *mariri* and I returned to sit in the chair, looking out over the night, alone with my thoughts.

Suddenly I felt a hand stroking my head and, looking up, I saw Susana standing there.

We clasped hands, the renewed contact flowing between us.

I took her in my arms and she curled into me, enfolding her warm back into my muscles and bones. Soft again. We held each other, each new movement surrendering and cherishing. We kissed and, looking in her eyes, they seemed to sparkle everywhere.

Then I felt the medicine within me, and I understood that I was a man with strong medicine, deep enough to hold us and to heal us.

As Susana and I left the maloca, Juan was singing again, a chant that seemed to contain all the joy of the awakening earth and home, of good things and ancient peoples.

Thank you, Maestro, I silently told him as I began my climb up the hill where Susana was waiting for me.

A couple of months into our stay at Mayantuyacu, I lay on my back beside the river in the little canyon, my head resting on the smooth stone, gazing into the blue-beyond-blue of a smoldering Amazon sky. The green of the leaves of the came renaco spread luminous above me, as if on the brink of bursting into emerald light. The air felt as clean as the inside of granite. From my vantage point, the world glowed, and nature operated serenely, cradling each thing in its place.

Yet no fit place could be found in the landscape of visions I was entering there. A tapestry was being woven whose strands I had yet to pass out of, through which, wandering in the world of spirit, I felt I perceived only fragments—or figments—of patterns.

Watching the green flight of a guacamayo and hearing its call from the canopy, I was aware I was not simply marking the passage of a parrot. The guacamayo is also the spirit of a tree, and its call, emerging out of the infinite unknown strands of the forest, carried information to those who had dieted the guacamayo caspi.

But then looking again there was just a parrot chattering away with its fellows on a branch. Many nights after ceremony, I lay gazing into the geometrical heights of the thatched roof of the maloca, wondering whether I were in an Incan temple in disguise, some structure of spirit more enduring than stone, more essential than its mere expression in time.

The tracks being laid down in my memory looked more and more like stumblings in the forest, yet they also followed a mysterious pattern, like the weaving stitchery of a Shipibo cloth. It had come to me the only way to discover this pattern was to walk it, blindly, as a labyrinth. Perhaps the thread of memory would serve as a rope to draw out some of the numinous power of that realm, to leave an imprint of the intelligence of plants, which I would eventually learn how to translate.

My life had become a virtual fast. No alcohol, beef or pork, salsas or spices. My sugar intake was limited to fruit, although sometimes we abandoned it for stretches, along with other stimulants like coffee, tea, and that enigmatic mineral, salt.

The weight had long fallen from my body. The droopy little ring I had once carried around my waist was long gone with the purges at Takiwasi, but in photos with curanderos taken during that time my face still had a cherubic plumpness to it—at least seen from the eyes of the very lean human being I had become.

Beyond feeling as substantial as a dried-up leaf, something was surfacing in my character I wasn't sure I wanted to see. Looking in the pocket mirror I traveled with, something spent, already withered at the stalk, gazed back at me in the light of my face. Shuffling and cautious, pedantic and grave, an old man had come to inhabit my movements and thoughts. White hairs sprang up on my head. The light in my eyes was wintry dim.

I studied myself. Was my spirit also fasting? Or was death closer to me?

Or by surrendering to the accelerated processes of birth and death in the plants, was I caught in their endless coil? I was dying, I figured. And I was choosing it. I wanted the life of the plants, their gift in me, their intelligence and connection with creation.

The choice seemed justified by the sublime moment of acceleration where, like an astronaut breaking free of earth's gravity, one floated free of the constraints of time and space into spirit. The experience could be subtle or barely navigable, blissful or harsh, but I felt compelled to master it.

Often, crouched like a cat by the turbulent edge of the river, my knees digging in to the hard rock and my head resting on my flattened palms, I would journey at the end of my sessions with ayahuasca, the seams between the worlds suddenly undone, all memory of having a body long gone. There I entered the archives of the plants, and I saw that the Incans are not lost because all their knowledge and culture is preserved— along with every other culture that has been on the earth—in the cellular memory of plants. But how to access it?

Other times I would suddenly pop into a space where all the curanderos, living and dead, gathered to consult over how to treat the diseases of the world. Voices would welcome me and compliment me for finding the way, but, just as in the case of the archives, the interior remained swathed in mist.

I would return to my incarnation genuinely surprised that among all the existences in the universe, I inhabited this particular one.*

My experiences were heady. I was Luke Skywalker exploring the Force. I was Neo learning the Matrix. *But if everything is so wonderful,* I asked, contemplating my hoary image in the mirror, *then why am I turning into Rip Van Winkle?*

How did I know I wasn't one of those characters governed by Neptune, willing to annihilate himself by worshipping other realms? I had no wish to be a lost poet, leaving behind fragmented immortal verses and a skeleton in the wilderness. I didn't mind having a savage light in my eyes, but only if it meant I could curl up with the other jaguars and sleep well into the jungle night.

The tension I was feeling reached its height one day when Susana sat down at the table with me where I was taking notes.

She was flourishing those days. The healing experiences the Maestro had promised had begun occurring, and she was busy conducting inter-

---

*James Hillman offers these highly relevant observations about dreams that explain much about the terrain encountered within the vine of the dead:

> *According to a Scandinavian school of ethnological research on soul (Arbman, Paulson, Hultkrantz), there is a world-wide experience of two kinds of souls, documented not only in the higher cultures of Homeric Greece, Ancient Egypt (Ka and Ba), China (hun and p'o), but continues to be found in this century among peoples who stretch across the great Asian land mass, from the Lapps on the Atlantic to Siberians facing Alaska, and then among American Indians as well. . . .*
>
> *This "dual pluralism" of soul . . . refers on the one hand to the life-soul that is multiple, having various associations with body parts and emotions, and so is called "body-soul," "breath-soul," and "ego-soul." On the other hand, there is a free-soul or psyche-soul . . . which is equivalent with and manifests as a "shadow-soul," "ghost-soul," "death-soul," "image-soul" . . . and "dream-soul." In Arbman's words, the "body-soul or -souls and the psyche-soul are independent of each other, have different natures and origins, as well as different tasks and spheres of activity." The psyche-soul "appears only outside the body" and, limited to this form of existence, "it is out of play in waking, conscious, and active states of the person," says Paulson. During these waking conditions, the psyche-soul is fully passive and no longer represents the personality as it does during dreams, visions, and shamanic trances.*[5]

views with her participants and transcribing them for analysis. Every day she was making more friends in the jungle around her, too. That morning I had found her with her work spread in front of her, absorbed in playing with a cute little insect that looked a cross between a lady bug and a spider. She introduced it to me as "buggy," and I watched how it kept climbing onto her like a pet and nestling itself onto the fabric of her sleeve as she tried to write. Now, fishing out her little pipe carved in the image of an owl, she lit it and sat back with a distant look in her eyes.

"I just had the funniest conversation with Henarte," she said.

Henarte was one of the workers, a tall, lean young man with a missing ear who was often seen tending the fires of the medicine kitchen. Like many of the workers, his childhood had been spent in the jungle. He was so in his element at Mayantuyacu that he chopped wood in his bare feet.

"Yes?"

"Well, he called you something very funny. You see, Mireya and I met him on the path from the shower and the subject of our ages came up. We told him we were nearly forty, and he didn't believe us, saying we looked so young. We laughed and told him you were almost forty too and he said you looked much older. We told him you're a gringo so your skin shows more wrinkles, but then he said you looked *gastado*."

"*Gastado?*" I asked, incredulous. That's a word used for a worn-out tire or shoe. It means "used up" or "wasted."

"Yes, isn't that funny?" she said. She took a deep draw off her pipe, and resumed gazing off at some distant place.

Gastado. I repeated the word to myself, and it sank into me like a depth charge. Then, to continue the ordinance metaphors, I went ballistic.

"Who the hell is this young punk to call me used up?" I demanded, a tremulous old man wielding his cane and threatening to thrash all comers.

Susana looked at me in shock. "I have no idea what he meant. I just thought it was funny. You're not gastado. Not in my eyes."

But I couldn't calm down. "Those are fighting words, where I come from," I declared. Susana's eyes widened further. *Should I challenge the young punk to fisticuffs? Perhaps a duel?* I found myself contemplating.

"Robert, relax. Henarte loves you. He didn't mean anything cruel with his words."

"No, he just called me gastado, is all," I retorted, and stalked out of the maloca.

Later Susana came and slid into my hammock. I had calmed down and was talking with Mireya, whose presence marked a release from the deep silence I had maintained for months with the unfamiliar world around. So while Tigrilla stalked the rafters above us, Mireya and I chatted about the world I used to inhabit, using concepts that fit my hands like old, familiar tools.

Susana politely changed the course of the conversation. She told me she had gone to Henarte to discuss my strong reaction to his calling me gastado. He had been very concerned.

"Robert thinks too much," she reported him as saying, paused in his work. "He should eat more papayas."

Papayas. . . . I should eat more papayas. . . .

"Can't I share anything in this bloody country without having it announced over a loudspeaker?" I demanded.

"Oh," Susana said.

"When I shared that with you, it was my own private process, not something meant for public consumption."

"Oh god, I'm sorry, Robert."

"That's the way the culture is down here, Robert," Mireya intervened.

"Well, I am not from this culture, and I need some space: my own life. I don't need everything I do and think broadcast like I'm the entertainment for the day. AND I AM NOT DYING!" I concluded, ineffectually slamming my fist on a stack of books beside me.

Tigrilla stopped her prowling and looked down from the rafters. A storm of giggling burst out in the kitchen.

Mireya and Susana were smiling. "You're definitely broadcasting now, Robert," Mireya said.

"Oh shit," I moaned, holding my head.

As my age continued its crab's march backward into senescence, strange intimations began reaching me from that other pole of mortality, the womb. They first surfaced in a nighttime reading of Edmund Spencer's Elizabethan romance *The Faerie Queene*.

Among Spencer's endless, immaculate lines of iambic pentameter, I encountered the walled-in garden of Venus, where clouds of teeming, naked infant spirits attend its gatekeeper, Genius, begging him to attire them in flesh:

> *Infinite shapes of creatures there are bred,*
> *And uncouth forms, which none yet ever knew,*
> *And every sort is in its sundry bed*
> *Set by itself, and ranked in comely row*
> *Some fit for reasonable souls to endow*
> *Some made for beasts, some made for birds to wear*
> *In endless ranks along arranged were*
> *That seemed the Ocean could not contain them there.*

A vision of the teeming thirst for incarnation, and the driving compulsion to be trapped in blind biological determinism, thrust into crushing growth processes as in a manufactory. Pierced by the image far out of proportion with its poetic worth, I closed the book and turned off my headlamp, telling myself that that was enough reading for one night.

The floodgates of memory broke a few nights later. In the session I saw the spirit of the tamamuri tree as Juan sang her as a *princesa,* a sirena. A beautiful pearly white throne, upon it a woman in white, serene and loving, burst upon my senses and was gone. Then something began jerking me about like a puppet, through the motions of receiving a soplada on my cupped hands and upon the top of my head, whipping away the darkness obscuring my vision. In a state of bemused wonder, I sat quietly until the Maestro began singing to the ayahuasca mariri. I left my mosquito net and drew closer. The call was unbearably compelling.

I sat in a circle of people already in deep concentration within the icaros, weaving sound back and forth among themselves. When the Maestro called me forward, I saw something greater than Juan sitting there. An ancient power had occupied his seat, venerable and sacred. I made a full prostration before this being, and I went forward to receive the healing.

As I sang with the Maestro for the first time, a braid of sound wove itself between him, Susana, and me, each strand enfolding the other and nourishing it onward. Asking the Maestro to sing a second time, I saw a realm of lost souls in my chest, a vast terrain, withered and ghastly, long deprived of light. A great golden radiance burst upon it, pouring in and restoring life. I needed to hear still more, and in my condition of mareación I could not find the words of the Shipibo icaro I loved. Attempting to offer an explanation, I raised my arms to imitate the flight of an eagle and found air filling my wings and I soared in flight. I sat before him riding the currents. . . .

"I want to learn how to fly," I told him.

"You're doing it," he said.

Overwhelmed by the vastness of the hawk's vision, I began to topple over onto my back, and the Maestro hastened to give me water.

We sat quietly a few moments. "Okay, you're ready," he said. I rose to return to my seat, but I was drawn in the direction of the river instead.

Standing at the entrance to the maloca, looking down into the landscape of agitated water, I saw a thing unveiled in the churning mist. Each step down the slope led ineluctably to the garden of rebirth. The spirits had gathered; the pathway to rejuvenation was lit. It was time to descend.

Keeping my footing through the vision, I made it down the final steps and sat on the stone beside the boiling current. A person dressed in white appeared on the rock beside me. Concentrating on the sound of flowing water, in a very short time I was drawn into a condition of desolate pain so absolute that not a single image could be associated with it, as if it came from before the time when images were made. Instead, a feeling of great antiquity and empty space.

As I wept, I felt someone holding me. Taking a moment to identify Brunswick and breathe one last time, I released all hold on the moment and dissolved into uttermost blackness.

I was back in the womb, and something had gone terribly wrong with my process of incarnation. A horror pure and boundless and unending—a great frozen echo of fear forever imprinted in my being.

Mireya heard the scream arising from the river. Scrambling across the mattresses, she went to Juan and said, "Maestro, can you sing?" The Maestro, coming out of concentration, began to sing.

I came to realizing I was wailing as Brunswick cradled my head and rocked me. "Let's go up," he said.

Managing to rise, I directed myself toward the maloca, but I discovered I had become an old man. My eyes were spent, my movements feeble and trembling, my balance gone. A psychology of dependency and shocked dismay at having been thrust into an old body was upon me. I tottered up, pushed by Brunswick from behind.

Setting me on the bench outside the kitchen, Brunswick left to fetch water and, returning, found me on my knees vomiting on the deck. He simply began pouring the water over my head. In the meantime, it had become circumstantially obvious I was before an altar in a church. Seeing the darkness in me and the light reaching in toward it, I knelt and clasped my hands in prayer at the bench, repeating, *"Gracias a Dios,"* over and over again.

Eventually, Brunswick was able to safely deposit me under my mosquito net and as I rested, comprehension began to coalesce out of the trailing ends of the vision. A spirit had intruded into the matrix of my development in the womb, parasitically inserting itself into my emerging consciousness. My natural course of development had derailed, and the terror I relived that evening had been of an uncomprehending fetus in the nurturing amniotic sea suddenly intruded upon by the demonic, finding its destiny abruptly mixed with a terrible other.

This had established the archetypal rift with the nurturing mother that was to be repeated in my later shelter experience, I saw. We automatically repeat the vast cruelties of our fate until we finally unravel it. Most paradoxical of all, I knew with certainty I had chosen to take on the intrusion before incarnation. *Why did I do that?* I asked myself, bewildered by the vertiginous opening of perspective. Why had I taken on such a nearly insurmountable task, suffering addiction and homelessness as a consequence?

It was out of love, the answer formed. Love for this spirit of disobedience that had to be tamed. Love for my little brother, who had died on the streets as such a young boy, whose karma had been too much for him to bear across lives. As best as I could make out, I had chosen to help him carry his cross by taking on a portion of his own battle of the soul.

And what gave me the possibility of unraveling this deep fate was that I took it on out of love in the first place.

Sitting with the Maestro and Susana in the early morning, the great insubstantial pageant faded, I told him about the powerful spirit I had seen in his body as I approached him for the healing that evening, calling it a bodhisattva, one of the great enlightened beings of the Buddhist tradition.

"Ah yes," Juan said. "He comes to me and inhabits my body, a very ancient man who spent many, many years walking the jungle."

"Who is it, Maestro?"

"I believe he is Moisés. . . ."

"Moisés?" I tried fitting the strange sounding word on my tongue. "Who is Moisés?" I asked, turning to Susana.

"Ummm, I think in English you say . . . Moses."

I don't know why I was still so easily stunned by such revelations. All I could think of saying was, "But Maestro, Moses was in the desert. . . ."

Juan smiled. "Ah yes, that's right. But it's the same thing."

"Maestro," Susana then asked, "if someone like Moisés, who died thousands of years ago, can still come and work with us, what is death?"

"Bueno, death is the profound dream of each person. So death is only a word for me. To die. Death. Because in itself one doesn't see death. For me, it would be only like an eternal rest, without using the word 'death.' Because I see that the spirits in rest, from there continue to work, working to help us who are living. So death, and I say this sincerely, is like a change, nothing more, of personality. We come only to be born in a body, in a form of reincarnation, to know the life of this world in which we find ourselves, to know the suffering, the struggle, to know the spirits of the living and also what we call death when we pass back into the world of spirit. From spirit we come and to spirit we return. So death, for me, is only a word, which I understand as a process of change in life.

"For that reason, ayahuasca helps us to die, because when we die, we encounter strong spirits. And in ceremonies with ayahuasca we may die and be reborn many times—we live, we die, we live, we die. And there are days when we encounter very strong spirits as well. So we have the opportunity to learn how to die with ayahuasca, to know death closely, what it is that is called life and death, life and death. Ayahuasca teaches us this, as well as how fear itself is death. To have fear is to be dying. Simply, you're dying. But if you conquer fear you are in the midst of life."*

A lively rollicking of spirits danced in my belly. In finally trailing the kaleidoscopic images of my visionary work back to their source, I had crossed some mysterious line and was now arrived, as if for the first time, in the rain forest. The pale, wintry light subsided in my eyes as the

---

*Juan's words illustrate a fundamental difference in approach to the ayahuasca experience, not only between Takiwasi and Mayantuyacu, but also between the conceptual paradigms of Europe and the indigenous world. Takiwasi, based as it is in the humanistic tradition and engaged in the necessary work of building up a healthy ego in the addict patients, constantly runs the risk of "performing a reductive operation" (in the words of James Hillman) upon the patient's visionary experiences through their interpretive methods of

> . . . reducing the eidolon, in which there is something archetypal, to a trait that can become part of my wholeness. This is indeed "growth"; but what grows is the ego, whose personality enlarges at the expense of the dream persons that it has become. In this subtle way . . . humanistic psychology . . . affords a psychological technique with which humanism can wipe out the last trace of its ancient enemy, the Gods, from their last retreat in the soul. Ever since Protagoras, all modes of humanism have tried to

harmony underlying our lives with the spirits, animals, and plants began to dawn. Strange intimations no longer appeared upon the surface of my mirror or in my bedtime readings.

A demonstration of the harmonious workings of the jungle was not long in coming, either.

---

maintain man in the center as the measure of all things. Now, by means of "subjective interpretation" or "Gestalt technique," the first and immediate experience of the mythic, which happens in dreams, can be put into the human beings as traits and parts of his nature. So, this mode of dream interpretation becomes just one more modern way of inflating the ego. The ideas of wholeness and creative growth cover the old hubris *of the* hero.

In contradistinction to the humanistic tradition, Juan states, "Death is the profound dream of each person," and "we have the opportunity to learn how to die with ayahuasca, to know death closely." As Hillman points out, "the old heroic ego loses its stuffing"[6] when the ability of death to instruct is admitted.

7 The Will to Heal Is the Will to Be Whole

The "reality" and "identity" of archaic
man was centered in sensuous self-
awareness and identification with a
close, ever-present and keenly sensed
world of nature: for us, our "self"
tends to be "realized" in a much more
shadowy, abstract, mental world. . . .
    This "objective" identity seems to
have been fully integrated into a cosmic
system that was at once perfectly sacred
and perfectly worldly. There is no
question that the Indian in the "sacred
city" felt himself completely at home in
his world and perfectly understood his
right place in it.

THOMAS MERTON

Anthropological reports of surgical work by shamans tend to focus on the garish and obvious. Like everyone else, I had grown up reading accounts of the witch doctor with his incantations and charlatan's trickery: the shaman is a "minister of the devil,"[1] and a "villain of a magician who calls demons,"[2] as some of the earliest priestly observers of the curandero's art wrote. Then along came the first rationalists to condemn them as "jugglers"[3] and "imposters"[4] deserving of "perpetual labor for their hocus-pocus."[5]

This trickster, working his gullible patients into a trance, would suddenly leap upon them and noisily suck the disease from the infected area, dramatically spitting out a wad of gore he had surreptitiously slipped into his mouth only moments before. Healings that occurred under such conditions were attributed to some sort of self-hypnosis on the part of the patient, and their accounts left the reader reveling in the fact that modern medicine was available just around the corner.

Never, during all my time in Brazil and Peru, had I witnessed such a questionable spectacle. It presented no problem to my rational intellect that Juan could treat different types of hepatitis, often with more success than Western medicine, because the work was based on plants and their molecular constituents, suggesting that the healing could be replicated if properly understood within the scientific methodology.

But at Mayantuyacu, I saw the greater scope of the curandero's art revealed, under circumstances that made it, if not exactly rational, intelligible. As if to set the stage, a couple of weeks earlier Juan had given us another of his "interview" accounts, in which he related his pilgrimage to the Andean highlands of Peru and his encounter with the spirits of the doctors of the Incas.

When I was a little boy I had a lot of fear of spirits. Even a little noise in my house was enough to make me cry out, "Mama, Mama, come and help me! It's the spirits of the dead!" My mother would bustle in, laughing, saying, "And what spirits do we have here?" and I would come back to my senses.

As time passed and I drank ayahuasca, I began conversing more and more with the spirits, although I was afraid of them. Sometimes when I heard the whistling of the souls, I would hide myself within the trees and watch the dead pass. It was like a game, but it wasn't. I feared they could do something to me, that they might kill me. But I persevered, and I continued to surpass my own fears. For that reason I can say that human beings can surpass themselves, can go beyond any condition. It's only in our manner of thinking that we are controlled by fear.

The place of the spirits of the Incas is called Makiwasi, the "Great House of the Spirits" in Quechua, a three-hour walk above the mountain village of San Pedro de Castas. At that altitude, you have to walk slowly, step by step, to control the beating of your heart. As well, the path is thickly hedged by San Pedro and other cacti with very sharp spines. If you go off the trail, you get jabbed. So we went carefully. It's very high, only sky and earth. You see nothing else, not even the peaks of other mountains.

I went with a friend, an Australian doctor, who had come with me to do the study, to know what the spirits of the dead are like.

When we arrived, bueno, for me it was a surprise to find the tombs of the dead. There were thousands and thousands of them that belonged to the empire of the Incas.

The first work I did with them was to go to seven tombs to talk with them, to ask them to keep an eye on me and protect me, especially from the evil spirits that could come against me.

Sometimes I found them in couples, no? Often I could see them because they had been thrown out of their tombs onto the earth. It is cold all the time, so they had only dried up and there they were: the man and the woman together.

Then we awaited the night. We slept below the rocks, because the rocks are like houses. And they are all filled with the dead. One has to clean out all the bones and spread out your bed to lie down. So my friend and I passed the first night beneath a rock, telling stories by the fire nearly all night because the cold was so intense.

❧

The place is the home of San Pedro. The Incas there drank and continue to drink San Pedro. Since there is no ayahuasca in that region, I brought a bottle of my own. But first I drank San Pedro to know the locale, how things were there. San Pedro and I saw each other, spoke together. And you know, San Pedro told me that each thing has its place. I'm of the jungle, San Pedro is of the mountains. So I don't drink San Pedro. I'm an ayahuasquero.

We passed nine days and nights with the Incas, with their spirits. In diet, concentrated, you know? Because we were alone, each of us, we would find our place and pass the day alone, as well as the night. There was only one hour during which we would meet together, and then we were on our own again.

When I first drank ayahuasca and concentrated myself, I called a spirit and a little bird came and flew around me, three times, and then left. I called, and it came. Then I said that I wanted to see the images of the gods—we were camped upon a plateau where one could lie back and look up into space. Looking above, I saw the images of all the gods appearing in the sky: Buddha, Christ, and Krishna. I could be in contact with them through the ayahuasca.

But my intention in going had been to abandon my fear and converse with the spirits of the dead Incas, because they were great men, very good doctors. The Incas knew how to operate on the brain. They made cures with plants, and when a person was sick with a tumor, they used plants to direct the operations. They worked as well with gold. When they made the incisions in the skull, they closed it with gold. These operations were very exact.

After I learned how to call Manco Capac, the chief of the first Incas, who began the culture, I could call all the other spirits of the dead Incas, because the chief directs all the members of the tribe. Then they came, appearing to me, and I asked them to teach me, to reveal how they healed their patients in that epoch. They taught me how to make the signs with my hands to indicate to the spirits where they should operate, in the brain or any other part of the body.

This was when I began to understand how to do spiritual operations.

In a spiritual operation, everything is as it is in life. The spirits of the doctors come and perform the operation when I call them, only they don't cut with a physical knife. They take out the part that is painful or infected, but they do it in the place it originates: the spirit. So the patient does not have wounds to heal afterward. They only have to remain in bed without moving for a day or so to stabilize themselves.

It was an amazing experience for me because I had never been in those regions with those studies, but it was my time to do them and make myself stronger, to center my studies in the Incas. All the spirits of the dead, and of our ancestors as well, are anxious to share their knowledge so they can work by extension in the world of the living. And they shared with me and taught me how to do the work they once had done, as well as how to use them for protection and to learn other spiritual things.

And I think best of all I no longer feared the dead. After this time with the dead, when I hear the spirits talking I say to them, "Hey! Come over here so we can talk. I'm your friend."

Carolina came hastening down the pillared avenues beneath the green vaulted ceiling like a fugitive upon the earth, rushing past the poor campesinos she encountered on the trail into Mayantuyacu with a curt *"Buenos días."* Her only goal was to get to her friend and ex-holotropic breathworker Susana who was somewhere out there in the mess of green.

One of those poor indios, beholding her face revolving between clear and half dark, said to himself, "She's come dying," and he watched her figure disappear over the next ridge. Turning to Brunswick, the Maestro sent him racing after Carolina but she would not slow and he could only point out the way.

At the sight of the cabins she accelerated further. Seeing her at the entrance to the big maloca, I tried to welcome her but she shot past me and ended up encountering Susana coming down the trail. Even then she kept her forward momentum and Susana grabbed her and said, "Stop! Where are you going? You've arrived!"

Carolina had come bearing what she believed could be a tiny death sentence buried deep in the center of her skull.

Some months before she had begun to suffer from migraine headaches of such intensity she would lose her sight, vomit, or go into convulsions. Medical tests revealed high glucose levels and decreased insulin production, indicating incipient diabetes, as well as altered hormone levels. Then an MRI revealed the presence of a microadenoma, a tumor less than ten millimeters in size, growing upon her pituitary gland, also known as the master gland of the body.

She began taking a chemical cocktail of medications and hormones to help the kidneys function, manage anxiety, and regulate glucose levels in her body, as well as to shrink the tumor, but she did not improve. Instead, she precipitously lost weight and suffered from severe depressive episodes. The doctors in her hometown of Santiago adopted a wait-and-see attitude, and they warned her if she did not show improvement in a few months they would need to operate, which meant burrowing into her head to remove the tumor.

The only referent remaining to Carolina when she reached crisis state was her faith in the therapeutic work of Susana. Her intuition told her that she needed to join her ex-therapist, even if it meant entering the jungles of Peru, as Susana suggested, to undergo treatment with a curandero. After consulting with her doctor, therefore, she set aside her medications and came to us.

Her first evening, she ended up lying in a hammock, vomiting from a migraine headache while Susana held her and Brunswick bathed her head with plants. She finally was able to go slip beneath her mosquito net and get some sleep at two in the morning.

The next day she awoke feeling better, and she felt herself beginning to decelerate. There was no sign of Susana. Carolina had breakfast and a shower, and then asked, "What's next?"

"*Nada,*" she was told. "Nothing." She began to get upset all over again.

She had come all this way and there wasn't even a schedule of activities to follow? Returning to her room, she rearranged her backpack, and wrote in her journal. After that, she had nothing else to do. It was eight o'clock in the morning. She was alone with herself for the first time in memory.

Carolina was in her late twenties, with black hair, dark eyes, and delicate white skin. When I first talked with her, she told me about the autistic children she worked with in the schools in Santiago, and about her boyfriend who had been in prison for years for conducting "terrorist" activities against the Pinochet regime. As we chatted, Tigrilla, who had developed an appetite for papaya, climbed up her leg to raid her plate. The cat stayed in Carolina's lap and took to visiting her cabin over the days that followed.

Unlike some visitors to Mayantuyacu, who came as disciples or for self-exploration, Carolina arrived with a concrete disease already defined within the parameters of Western science. We, on the other hand, had been working toward a preliminary sketch of the methods of Juan, and we were in a position to watch her healing process from an angle unavailable to those early anthropologists roughing it among their witch doctors.

The Maestro began her treatment gently with *agua icarada,* water he gave her to drink after he had sung and blown tobacco over it. Along with baths of ajo sacha, basil, and other plants, he prescribed long periods for her to sit by the river, absorbing the steam rising from it. As Carolina's system gradually detoxed, she began drinking two liters of paico tea a day to help her brain function and heal her internal wound, and later a stiff shot prepared from the roots of mucura to build up strength, as well as other medicinal plants such as came renaco and chuchuwasi. Following the initial severe migraine she experienced upon entering Mayantuyacu, her headaches never recurred.

Around her fifth day, right around the time she estimates the medicines had left her body, the insects moved in. They came like a militia of little doctors bearing syringes, and after initially being bitten only a few times a day, she began to suffer from hundreds of bites. She soon appeared like a burn victim, swathed in cloth over her entire body, even to the tips of her fingers—leaving only the half moon of her face revealed. She resisted using chemicals to treat it. Something told her the insects were allies, just like the water and the plants of Mayantuyacu, and that they were acting upon her body to get the disease out. But when she could no longer sleep for the torrent of bites coming from her mattress, we treated it with the most lethal insecticide we could find and left it in the sun for the day. It had no effect whatsoever.

As the pummeling went on, she began to surrender. She faced the fact that her skin was becoming deformed and at a certain point she asked, "What is it I have to learn from this wounded body?" She saw her body had become ugly, but it was just a body, nothing else. There was something more important than smooth white skin.

She began accustoming herself to doing nada. But nothing was a lot, really. She explained, "Do nothing transformed into thinking about Carolina and centering myself and listening to what I really wanted; to order my ideas." As she further decelerated, she beheld the silvering of the jungle under the moon one evening, and she asked herself, "For whom is this light? What am I supposed to learn from this night?" After that she lit her lamp very rarely in the cabin. "If it's night, it's supposed to be night," she said.

"I learned that in life we don't necessarily know whether something is good luck or bad luck," she told me. "I am here, now, and it is the now that is to be enjoyed. We are supported by something greater, and what must come to pass will pass." She began giving thanks for the tumor, because it taught her "there are people that love me, that I am alive, and that I need to listen . . . and there are other folks who I should not allow to come so close to me and my life."

She also began heeding the counsel of the Maestro, who told her, "Ask the spirit of the stones by the river to give you strength. Ask the plants to give you their wisdom." When Brunswick took her for a walk, she would request permission to embrace all the medicinal trees he introduced her to, and she embraced them all. To her it seemed as if she spent many hours walking in the forest, when really it had been only a few. She felt so tiny, so content with her place in creation: "The trees had carried on for millions of years with their wisdom and I would get preoccupied about what I was going to wear the next morning? It gave me a lot of peace, and peace about the tumor I carried in my head."

Insight into the deep interrelatedness existing within nature began to come to her. "There was lots of heat, lots of sweat. One day I asked, 'Oh, come, breeze, to refresh me,' and that night a strong breeze arose and everyone said, 'Oh, this is not ordinary.' "

At a certain point during her twenty-one days with us, the sensation came to her that she no longer had the tumor. "But it was only a sensation, there was nothing more solid to back it up."

"Treatment begins gently with the calling of spirits," said the Maestro, "the studying of what plants are required." Above all, Juan saw that Carolina needed the purified water of the river, and from the first moment he gave her *agua icarada,* water over which he had sung and blown smoke.

On her second evening, Carolina joined a ceremony. She understood nothing of the Maestro's icaros until she approached his seat for an individual healing. At that moment, while he sang and blew smoke over water in the same little cup that he served ayahuasca from, everything became crystal clear to her. We, on the other hand, were only aware how focused his icaros were on the spirits of space (as Juan calls God, Jesus, Buddha, and other divine spirits).

What Juan was doing was entering into concentration, invoking and ordering the arrival of the divinities for the moment of Carolina's operation. He was especially invoking the Sumiruna, the greatest doctor of the water, and his followers, as well as other curanderos who would assist him in the operation. Juan had decided that Carolina's condition was so grave that he needed to conduct an operation immediately. The work had to be rapid and precise; such an operation cannot be done twice, and is dangerous. That evening, directing the operation with the hand gestures he had been taught by the Incans, the spirits appeared to him as doctors wearing gloves and handling the same instruments used in a modern operating room.* He directed the cut to Carolina's brain and took out the disease.

---

*There are times when one wonders who is imitating whom across the frontier of spirit and matter.

Just as in literal surgery with a knife or laser, little is certain after such an operation. The system has to stabilize, accept the therapeutic intrusion, and reestablish itself upon new parameters in the aftermath. "The plants cure, but slowly. Time is necessary to heal," Juan said. But he had taken the first major step toward Carolina's healing, and it is perhaps notable that her migraines vanished after that night. The Maestro did not, however, relax, nor did he consider the process complete.

The experience of ayahuasca was "peculiar," said Carolina.

Initially, Juan did not want to give her the plant. She was a foreigner, and in grave condition. *Remedios suaves,* gentle remedies, was what he believed she required, but eventually Carolina asked to drink ayahuasca while participating in the ceremonies. "Her body wanted the plant," he said, and he acquiesced to give her a very mild dosage.

The first time she drank ayahuasca as well as agua icarada she fell asleep to the lightning blazing out of the jungle canopy. She slept profoundly, then awoke, and then slept again. Finally she entered concentration at a moment when Juan began to sing. She felt a sudden pressure in her chest and didn't know if she was going to vomit or not.

"Cry, cry little princess," Juan sang, and she began to cry, and then wept disconsolately. Saliva, mucus, and tears all came from her at once, in a sharpness of pain that almost made her cry out. Susana, sent by the Maestro, appeared, took her hand, and, sitting close beside her, sang icaros until the Maestro called Carolina forward and gave her a soplada. At this point Carolina felt that the pain had passed. Afterward her chest felt very open, giving her a sensation of being uncovered, and without protection.

As the day of Carolina's departure approached, she began to appear renewed. Her eyes had changed. They sparkled more and showed more self-possession. "The truth is, I delivered myself over to the experience immediately upon arriving. The anger was gone when I left, and when the Maestro told me I had come back to life, I felt it too. I had a second chance at life, and I left the jungle happy."

In her final ceremony with ayahuasca the Maestro called the spirits of the dead. As he sang, she felt a desire to dance and then she began to see spirits dancing about her. Opening her eyes, there was only the darkness of the maloca, but closing her eyes, everything came clear. People turned about her. She saw members of her family who had passed away—her brother and cousin and grandmother. They danced beside other spirits who she felt were doctors. They wove protection around her.

The Maestro said, "I am going to sing an icaro for the spirits of the animals," and her own animals began to appear to her, the ones she had had as a child. "There was my dog and my cat. I was so happy to see them again, dancing around me! And then there was another spirit that came to protect me, like the smoke of mapacho. It came and entered me, just like the animals."

She was very content and, upon returning to her cabin, she felt very protected. Afterward, when we met in Santiago, she told me, "Now, whenever I feel upset and anxious, I smoke a mapacho and blow smoke on myself and I feel again the spirits protecting me and I calm down. Everything is going to be okay."

Carolina's departure from Mayantuyacu was very different in character than her arrival; there were hugs all around for everybody. Even so, the Maestro took a conservative stance and told us he believed she would need to return for further treatment. She was off to face the final, and perhaps most difficult, stage of the healing process—integration. It was all well and nice to have had sweet dreams in the jungle, but could she transplant the new Carolina into the old environment? We had already seen the treatment of a few addicts at Takiwasi go astray at this final stage. Unable to resist the pull of the disintegrative forces in their families and their social milieu, they had relapsed back into addiction.

To make matters worse, the burden of the integration stage lies nearly entirely with the returned pilgrim. Who is to guide the fresh initiate in their process of contextualizing the raw experience of the medicines? Blank stares, incomprehension, doubts, or even dismissals are the daily fare. A step beyond these initial reactions lie the inadequate models of interpretation and deeply held cultural prejudices against immersion in nature.

Healed or healer, this is the line over which many fail to carry the medicine.

The earliest modern European initiate into native ways of healing that we know of was the conquistador Alvar Núñez Cabeza de Vaca.[6] Shipwrecked on Galveston Island, he made an enforced pilgrimage, along with two companions, through the Rio Grande valley and then back south into Spanish Mexico between 1528 and 1536. Befriended by native tribes and following trails already etched upon the landscape, he received his initiation after losing his way and "spending several winter nights sleeping naked in a pit in the Texas desert under a north wind,"[7] an experience very much in the tradition of the vision quest. Upon recovery, he had a "knack for healing."[8] Word spread of the marvelous doctor wending his way south, and tribes eagerly welcomed his arrival, bringing forth their sick for him to pray over.

Ironically, upon Cabeza de Vaca's arrival in Mexico and the resumption of his previous identity as a civilized Spaniard, he lost his healing powers. Unable to integrate his two identities, one founded in the dream-time of nature and the other in the artifice of his European background, he lost not only the ability to heal, but, as Gary Snyder suggests, "the *will* to heal, which is the will to be whole."[9] For Cabeza de Vaca, there were "real doctors"[10] in the city, and he began to doubt the powers that had mysteriously come to him.

This is the dilemma and the agony of the pilgrim's return: "To resolve the dichotomy of the civilized and the wild, we must first resolve to be whole."[11]

This resolution can be far more demanding than the pilgrim imagines. It constitutes the rigorous work of a lifetime.

Carolina's impression upon returning to Santiago was of the absence of natural grace in her old world, as well as excess and contamination in that environment. When her mother welcomed her home by serving her a cola, Carolina couldn't drink it. Her room was filled with things she didn't need, and she was shocked to acknowledge that her bathroom, off which was located a room where she cleaned herself and eliminated wastes, was virtually in the same room where she prayed: "In the jungle, you do your business at a distance from where you live." It was then, she told me, that she learned the difference between poverty and humility.

"In the jungle, I had a bed and a candle, and that was sufficient. I am clear to be poor doesn't mean to not have. The people of the jungle are super-humble, but they aren't poor, because they have everything in abundance. The fruit, the water, the air, the oxygen, is abundant. They are not poor. To be humble, simple, is not the same as being poor."

The torment with the physicians and their battery of tests began. "I used to like the exams for diabetes, because they gave me sugar, but this time the exam wouldn't work because I vomited the sugar back up. They had to test me twice, and then I had to rest for hours in order to have the strength to get home." An injection of radiated iodine was worse, leaving her extremely sick. Finally, the ordeal over, she began her period of awaiting the results of the tests.

In the meantime, she carried the forest like a crystal within her. She returned to church, "Not to follow the routines but to have space to pray," and her sense of connection with community spontaneously reasserted itself. Content with her life, with the same ups and downs, she faced them by posing a question: "Who knows if this is good or bad?"

Traveling for a month, she attended a wedding of friends in Panama, relegating her health concerns to the same emotional region as the forest she bore within her. Upon her return, she found a fat envelope set prominently upon her bed—the results of the hospital exams.

Taking it up in her hands, she turned it about. Had her time at Mayantuyacu been something more than an idyllic dream? Praying hard, she broke the seal and pulled out the contents.

There was no trace of a tumor.

She read it three times. The entire area affected—the pituitary gland and the structure of the brain—had all completely returned to normal. Blood tests were within normal range. She was healed.

She gave thanks to all, even to the insects.

Returning to meet with her physician, she handed him the results. He looked them over and then at her as if he couldn't believe it.

"What did you do?" he asked her, visibly affected.

"Nothing," she replied. "I drank water."

"But what water?"

"Water from a river, tea of paico, some preparations of plants . . ."

Her physician took a colleague aside, showing him the exam results and saying, "Look, this patient had a tumor in March, and now it's gone. . . ."

A few months later, at the end of our interview, she raised her hands in a gesture of helplessness and asked me, "How do you explain to people that to heal yourself you drank tea of paico, bathed with a plant, and took steam baths?"

Carolina continues without remission, and without any need for medication.

Carolina's healing demonstrated something elegantly simple, at least to us as amateur participant-observers. Healing comes from reembedding the patient into a living cosmology, a hierarchy of being that supports and gives meaning to their process of living and dying. The cure, therefore, did not lie in removing the tumor. In fact, in what occurs as paradoxical to Western medicine, her real healing might have lain in the *dying* of the tumor—as long as her death process was her path back to life.

A remarkable account of the role of nature in death processes is given by psychologist Victor Frankl in his classic narrative of his experiences in the Auschwitz concentration camp:

> *This young woman knew that she would die in the next few days. But when I talked to her she was cheerful in spite of this knowledge. "I am grateful that fate has hit me so hard," she told me. "In my former life I was spoiled and did not take spiritual accomplishments seriously." Pointing through the window of the hut, she said, "This tree here is the only friend I have in my loneliness." Through that window she could see just one branch of a chestnut tree, and on the branch were two blossoms.*

"I often talk to this tree," she said to me. I was startled and didn't quite know how to take her words. Was she delirious? Did she have occasional hallucinations? Anxiously I asked her if the tree replied. "Yes." What did it say to her? She answered, "It said to me, 'I am here—I am here—I am life, eternal life.'"[12]

But Carolina didn't need to take that route. Her embracing of the trees in the forest probably did as much to heal her as any of the plants she drank or any of the rituals conducted by Juan. I dare say it fulfilled one of the deepest needs of our souls: to live in a reciprocal universe, a benevolent order in which, when we call out, we are resoundingly heard. This, I now believe, is the true basis of shamanism.

The Japanese have a form of therapy akin to what Carolina had undergone. They call it *shinrin-yoku,* wood-air bathing, and they have devoted entire symposiums to the benefits of wood-air bathing and walking. Japanese researchers as well have discovered that "when diabetic patients walk through the forest, their blood sugar drops to healthier levels."[13] Joan Maloof goes on to note in her *Teaching the Trees: Lessons from the Forest* that researchers "working in the Sierra Nevada of California found 120 chemical compounds in the mountain forest air—but they could only identify 70 of them,"[14] and she speculates that "the trees may be altering our perceptions with their chemicals. The volatile molecules evaporate into the air and come into contact with the sensory neurons in our nasal passageways. The olfactory nerves send messages directly to the limbic system in our brains."[15] Edible monoterpenes, produced by pine trees, have been shown by research to both prevent and cure cancer, and they are used in many chemotherapy drugs. However, there is not a scrap of research into whether the compounds given off by trees are also monoterpenes. Maloof goes on to ask is this because "forest air cannot be patented, and consequently no money is to be made from it?"[16]

January 21, the Maestro's deadline for delivering to Susana sufficient healing experiences for her study, had come and gone. And while she had conducted in-depth interviews with participants from North America, Brazil, and Argentina who reported having their worlds turned inside out by the Maestro's icaros, she had yet to collect all her data. In the midst of plenty, it would have been niggardly to complain of lack. But still, the omission nagged at us. It wasn't like Juan to miss the mark in such matters.

So we inquired discreetly, "Maestro, what happened with the healing experiences? Wasn't the study supposed to be completed on the twenty-first?"

"I don't know," he said, shrugging his shoulders. You can never tell with spirits, he seemed to be saying.

Then word reached us that one of the workers at Mayantuyacu had been hospitalized in Pucallpa for a virulent outbreak of symptoms that had left the doctors wagging their beards in recognition: witchcraft. They were just in the process of explaining to her she needed a shaman, not a doctor, when Juan arrived to take the worker home and bathe her with plants. Her fever and pain immediately subsided. Stabilized, she contacted Susana, who recorded her peculiar tale.

During the ayahuasca session a few evenings previous, the Maestro had sung a dart carved of fish bone out of her foot, a piece of brujería she had been carrying in her system since she had worked among native tribes on the border of Peru and Brazil many years before. At the height of her mareación, ayahuasca had told her it was going to take the dart out, but the reaction of her system would be so intense that she might die.

"I don't care," she replied. "Take the thing out of me."

So the Maestro had drawn the jagged thing out of the bottom of her foot. Wrapping the bloody dart in tissue, he had it taken down to the river and cast it into the boiling water.

Juan had delivered the concluding healing experience after all.

The fieldwork portion of the study was drawing to a close and Susana and I packed up our bags and returned to Pucallpa for her to conduct her final interviews before returning to Mayantuyacu to complete our work.

There were then two goals foremost in our minds. The first was to resolve the dilemma of what to do with our little cat when we left South America for the United States. Tigrilla had flourished in the jungle, and we did not know if we could transplant her to an urban environment in America, or if she could survive the immigration process with her unique character intact. We loved her and did not want to flatten her spirit and make her into a neurotic housecat. But if we left her, she would be alone, a little malnourished cat fighting it out among the chickens for food scraps. Who would treasure her like we had? Who would journey with her like we had?

So we attempted a minor expedition. As we hiked the entire way out of Mayantuyacu in the stifling heat, Tigrilla valiantly loped by my side, and arrived at the river panting to burst. She then faced the ordeal of the launch taking us downriver. When we made Honoria, she was disassociated, and by the time we boarded the packed vehicle for Pucallpa, she was *tharn* as Richard Adams once put it. When we stopped momentarily to pick up other passengers, she leaped from my lap out the window and disappeared into a field of high grass. Everyone unloaded, and the driver put on his finest long-suffering face in light of these foreigners with their cat. Wading into the grass, a small group of us fanned out, calling her, but there was no response. Finally halting, I told myself, "This cat and I are connected. I can find her if I just get still and concentrate." Taking a moment to collect myself, I looked down and found her curled up in a ball at my feet.

In the hotel room in Pucallpa, Tigrilla acted like a little android disconnected from her master program. She went feral, climbing the walls and clawing and biting Susana. By the time the interviews were completed, Susana and I were completely flummoxed. How were we to continue true to our connection to this cat we cherished? Tigrilla's future with us remained uncertain.

Turning our attention to our second goal, we began preparing to return to Mayantuyacu. There we would take the radical step of abandoning all ties with the world and enter the deep jungle to do a traditional diet in the style of the shamans of old.

8 A Sweet Odor Shall Enter Their Bones

When Rama sat, facing the east, Viswamitra taught him the mantras to summon the occult weapons. The rishi himself had the astras from Siva, long ago, when he was still a king and had need of them. When Rama spoke the secret mantras, the lords of the astras appeared before him. They were neither of this world nor yet in the next: they stood between realms, their bodies of pristine light. The eyes of some were turquoise flames; others had locks of green tongues of fire.

They said to Rama, "Now we are your slaves; we will do your bidding, whenever you want."

Rama said to them, "Dwell in my mind, until I have need of you."

THE RAMAYANA

After many months rubbing shoulders with practitioners of curanderismo, we had come to distinguish what we called the three pillars of Amazonian shamanism: purging, work with psychoactive plants, and dieting.

Each of these practices is distinct, while at the same time mutually interpenetrating and supporting. At Takiwasi, for example, with its strong focus on cleansing the body of toxins accumulated from drug addiction, ceremonies with the purgative yawar panga are as frequent as work with ayahuasca. Yet purging often occurs spontaneously in ceremonies with ayahuasca, the psychoactive component of the triad.

Dietary restrictions, of course, are pervasive. With shamanism's credo that the body *is* spirit, or "the temple of God," to use the old saw, it followed that you didn't eat just anything. As in many religions, there were food taboos: it had been months since I had last sipped a glass of wine, flavored food with Tabasco sauce, or eaten red meat.

True diets, however, were performed for more mysterious ends, and, needless to say, they had nothing in common with weight-loss programs.

In "dieting" a plant, the suppliant takes the plant into her body, receiving its virtue and blending spirits in a mutual exchange clear across the phylogenetic tree—an exchange essentially identical to working with ayahuasca, but differing in depth and duration. It was the profundity of communion that comes from dieting that lay behind Sandra's enigmatic words the first evening we met Juan: "I often can't tell if it's him or a plant that is talking."

Plants that are dieted have *madres,* strong healing or teaching spirits. We lived surrounded by these plants in the jungle and they formed part of the lore of our daily lives: ajosquiro, lupuna, ayahuma, chullachaqui caspi, tamamuri. These trees sheltered us and towered above us, spreading their arms to contain the life of the jungle and sky. They were powerful doctors and subtle teachers, comprising the ancient libraries and Internet systems of the native peoples of the world.

I already had some experience with dieting: came renaco for my back, camalonga for protection against witchcraft, carrizo to teach me to sing.

But these were done in relatively populated conditions. Traditional diets are conducted in deep jungle, in total isolation from human contact.

I could already visualize our lives to come in detail.

We had already visited the tambos where we would diet: two little dwellings facing each other across a confluence of two streams, high enough above the canyon so that when the floods came they would not be swept away. Floors of thick slices of bark, struck off the tree like rind and pressed flat, lay upon a platform of sectioned logs and posts set in the earth. Roofs of pure palm frond, secured with strips of husk upon simple A-frame structures. Wooden bed frames had been hauled the entire distance and set there for the comfort of patients, upon which lay simple, thin mattresses and fresh sheets under mosquito nets. A hammock strung up between the two main supports of the structure synched the whole tambo up tight whenever someone lay in it. A little shelf suspended by string from the roof would hold my bottles of medicine and my altar to Saint Francis.

Along with total isolation would come extreme renunciation of food intake, beginning with salt* and continuing on to cover a spectrum of sugars, proteins, and vitamins. A pile of green bananas, a bag of rice, and a

---

*Jacques Mabit, in a lecture in Paris in 2003, spoke about the role of this enigmatic mineral in traditional Amazonian diets, and offered these speculations about its role in the life of civilized man:

> In the history of humanity, one notices that the routes of salt are identical to the routes of high civilizations, whereas animals in the forest do not consume salt, or very little. Now salt plays a role as electric or energetic isolator. We have introduced salt into our diet to permit us a certain degree of separation from nature, whereas animals keep directly in touch with nature. They feel nature, and a wild animal to whom one gives salt begins to become docile and you can tame it more easily because it loses its reflexes and its sensitivity to the calling of nature. We have inversely won a relative distance from nature, which gives us a certain degree of freedom in comparison with animal impulses, and allows us more opportunity to choose. Therefore, salt introduces a dimension of culture by releasing us from the imperatives of nature. Salt seems thus to be linked to the birth of the individual and free will.
>
> Now the excess of salt plays a leading role in hardening the arteries, particularly those of the heart and the brain, just as our distance from nature makes us lose our connection with our nature, with the spirit of things and life. Thus, salt has a very important function and eating without salt represents a kind of regression, which like any

stack of brown roots of yucca would make up our weekly fare. Twice a day we would kindle a fire against the wetness and cook rice and tea in the soot-coated pots, singe the peels of the bananas until black, and then lay their bared white flesh against the flames until they were toasted fine. We would fetch water from the thermal springs downstream, forking out with a stick any boiled snakes that had accumulated, and wash our pots in the stream below, counting the *patitos,* the little ducklings Brunswick had released there, to make sure no cruising wildcats had eaten one of their number.

Ah, the ascetic life. I was eager for it, and I feared it. The prospect of hunger loomed like a cold storm front on the horizon.

That evening we sat with the Maestro in Mayantuyacu and devised the regimen of our diet, choosing the plants that would be our companions for a month. Susana and I were unanimous in wanting to drink tobacco, whose characteristics as an establisher of boundaries, a director of plants, and a protector and purifier were reminding me more and more of Hermes, the messenger spirit of medicine, thievery, and boundaries who once allied himself with the traveler Odysseus.

We also both chose mucura, an unprepossessing little plant, whose roots, when soaked in water, make a fiery tonic to strengthen the body.

The Maestro prescribed shihuahuaco—another *"¡dispara bien!"* plant—that he claimed developed the capacity for shamans to calibrate their energy and fire accurately, as well as chuchuwasi for protection and vitality.*

---

regression is potentially dangerous. However, within the context of ritual, the regression is temporarily allowed because it aims to heal. The absence of salt reduces the electrical projections of the body and makes the subject temporarily vulnerable to "opening" his energetic body. As well, the intensity of the psychic and sensorial perceptions of the subject requires a protective isolation in a silent and undisturbed area.

It is then obviously necessary to "close" the energetic body so that on leaving isolation in nature the induced hyper-sensitiveness goes down.

If you brought a wild animal to the Place de la Concorde, you would make it mad.[1]

*Chuchuwasi is also popularly used as an aphrodisiac to increase the capacity for straight shooting in another context.

Then he gave us a bottle to sip that he had brought to the table with him. Its contents tasted a little like root beer. Susana and I looked at each other, pleasantly surprised.

"What plant is this, Maestro?"

"Bueno, that is Shihuahuaco." He lit a mapacho and blew the smoke over himself. "The Shihuahuaco has a spear of steel and can help you also in the hunt. Sometimes the spirit comes while you are dieting, hands you the spear, and shows you what to shoot at. If you miss, your diet is not going well and you have to diet longer. If you hit, the assessment is good."

Susana, who was now a seasoned veteran at dieting, chose to continue communing with the queen of the forest, chacruna. I chose to drink chullachaqui caspi, the lord of the forest whom Brunswick introduced me to the day we went to harvest the came renaco.

Returning to our cabin, I flipped open the moldering text of the Book of Enoch that always accompanied us and my eyes fell on this passage:

Among these there was a tree of an unceasing smell; nor of those which were in Eden was there one of all the fragrant trees which smelt like this. Its leaf, its flower, and its bark never withered, and its fruit was beautiful.

I exclaimed; Behold, this tree is goodly in aspect, pleasing in the leaf, and the sight of its fruit is delightful to the eye. Then Michael, one of the holy and glorious angels who were with me, answered,

And said; Enoch, why dost thou inquire respecting the odour of this tree? Why art thou inquisitive to know it?

Then I, Enoch, replied to him, and said; Concerning everything I am desirous of instruction, but particularly concerning this tree.

And that tree of an agreeable smell, not one of carnal odour, there shall be no power to touch until the period of the great judgment. This shall be bestowed on the righteous and humble. The fruit of this tree shall be given to the elect. The sweet odour shall enter into their bones.

Everything seemed propitious. We made our final preparations to enter the jungle the following morning and fell asleep to its humming and chirruping, content to enter even more deeply into its heart.

The next morning we lost our spirit cat.

Stowing the very last items and tightening the straps on our backpacks, we were at the point of fetching Tigrilla and departing when a woman came walking up the path, her head down and her brow furrowed.

"Tigrilla just died," she told me, looking up at me with glassy eyes.

I looked at her in disbelief. At the very juncture of going into a traditional diet, after months of preparation, we had lost our ally, our little one?

Racing down the hill, we found her limp body lying on the deck of the maloca outside the storeroom. She had chosen at the last moment to consume a little plate of rice the Maestro had left in a corner. It was laced with rat poison and Brunswick had been unable to administer the antidote in time. Susana and I collapsed on the deck beside her, taking her into our hands and caressing her, calling her name in disbelief that this vital force had ceased.

Why had she done it? Traits of feral independence had been competing with her bond with us, but each time we returned from Pucallpa and another minor abandonment, we had drawn her back in. But her wildness had been getting stronger. Just the day before, instead of sitting by her food bowl and looking up at me in polite request, she had swatted off the top that kept the ravenous insects out of it. As we both watched the top rolling on the floor, I took in the implication. The jungle was no joke for a little cat, and if we could not be there for her consistently she would do what she needed in order to survive.

Watching us once again packing, and packing so thoroughly that nothing remained in our cabins, had she come to the conclusion that now she had to truly fend for herself and gone foraging farther than anyone could have expected? Or had she chosen this way of poison, like the Little Prince?

Through a haze of tears, Susana and I gently cleaned the vomit off her face and the feces off her rear legs and tail. Carrying her up the hill, we sat with her on our laps on the front steps, stroking her fur in the golden sunshine, telling her how she would always live in our hearts.

The truth was, Tigrilla had never been our pet.

She was our ally, and we were involved in a deep interspecies communication with her. Evolving together, she had scrambled like a little monkey through our ayahuasca visions, taught us middle ways through our inner blockages, sat guardian on top of our mosquito nets, and reduced us to the joyful, helpless laughter of little children.

As she reached from the rafters when I came in from a ceremony one night and delicately placed the soft of her paw upon my cheek, I saw expressed through all of her frame a love like that of a mother for a child, and a child for her father, and an angel for the one she is watching over.

Who was this cat who joined us as we learned to move through this terrain of spirits? Who had so many intelligences evolving within her?

The blow was terrible. We had to place our love into the earth.

Choosing a spot beneath a *piñon colorado,* a small tree with velvet-smooth deep green leaves and red flowers sacred to El Señor de los Milagros, we dug a hole in the soft earth with a machete. Carefully curling her up and wrapping her in a Shipibo cloth, I placed my prayer beads in with her, pressing their carved image of a hummingbird silhouetted against a crescent moon against her heart. Susana put in a Tibetan ornament, a symbol of protection for her journey, and we interred her.

As we gently covered her with earth, I hoped an archaeologist would come along and find her three thousand years later and say, "These were a people who truly loved their cats."

In the fading light of the day we gathered up our last necessities and began the walk back to the tambos. Following the path along the river, I could half see the fleet form of Tigrilla accompanying us, leaping the boulders and hopping the crevices, just as she had always done.

In my dream, the jungle is looming and dark, the earth spongy and watery beneath my feet, falling away into crevasses and depressions. Vines and fronds, tendrils and branches consume me, bearing me down. Entangled in a huge vine, I am absorbed into an ominous weight, a massive wet tree. Fighting desperately, I tear myself free and awake in a morning dark from the blanket of rain cloud covering the landscape.

As I reached for my flashlight in order to record the dream in my journal, thunder sounded like a warning drum. We were a week and a half into our diet.

Even as I wrote, the rain arrived, an inundation so powerful it amazed me yet again that the finely woven carapace of palm frond just over my head continued to shield me. Rising from my bed, I walked teetering to the edge of the tambo and peered out. Breakfast would be late this morning. The river and its tributary stream were already rising and I would soon be cut off on top of my little hillock, alone. Lighting a mapacho, I blew smoke over my medicines, drinking them one by one, and then settled down to watch the river precipitously rise.

All that morning I watched logs the size of whales float by below me, all the gentle curves and drops of the river consumed by the blind unleashed torrent. I sat remembering through a haze of melancholy my distant home in the Sierra Nevada and the friends left far behind.

Hours later, single drops of water now delicately falling from the tips of my palm frond roof, I leapfrogged across the swollen stream and climbed the hill up to the kitchen. Susana was there, fanning the flames of the little fire she had kindled, and she offered me a cup of Carrizo tea. Sitting on a tarp, I related to her my dream of escaping the devouring tree.

She caressed me and said, "Next time, surrender to the vine. It won't hurt you to become a tree."

As I sat sipping my tea I thought to myself that we really have no idea of the incredible array of sensorial experiences we provide ourselves by eating—until we go cold turkey, that is, and live like the rest of the creatures of the planet, who live off the strictly limited nutritional resources of their ecological niche: foods without spices, unprepared, unvarying. After days of green banana, the very idea of a spaghetti dinner, a strip steak, a pizza, even a simple roast chicken breast with salt, or that shimmering grail of alimentation—a cup of coffee—seemed overwhelming explosions of mood- and mind-altering sensorial gratification.

Our diet was paralleling the fasting of our other senses as well. Each day, three times a day, we drank waters prepared with the barks or roots of different trees and plants, waters with different flavors and punches. They passed through my body like the streams passed through every part of the landscape, like the rains fell from above, like the murmuring presence of water passed ceaselessly through my senses of sight, hearing, smell, and touch.

In withdrawal, even the things of civilization with their meaningless sensorial overloads—malls, freeways, and the media—had taken on an allure in my dreams. Sometimes they danced before me like sylphs, perhaps because they were complexities I understood. Perhaps a native of the Amazon would feel equally bereft of familiar referents sitting in a shopping mall, I speculated, and would dream of trees.

"Bito, I woke up last night and the spirits were doing an operation on me," Susana said, breaking into my thoughts.

"Well, how was it?" I asked, not knowing what to expect.

"I woke up and felt needles placed in very precise locations on my body. They were giving me a transfusion from the power of the river, and I felt guilty because I was *supposed* to be dreaming. Dream was my anesthesia, and I had stumbled into something I wasn't supposed to see."

Sipping our tea, we took in the jungle surrounding us.

"Even as I try to describe it, I can feel it turning into words and the experience passing away. But I feel so grateful. . . ."

We sat silently for a time. "They're so impeccable," she concluded.

The Maestro came to visit that afternoon and sat resting the blade of his machete against the inside of his left boot while we conversed. We talked of the river waters, of their rise and fall, of their sound that accompanied us day and night at the tambos like music. Susana said in the sounds of the water and the jungle she could hear a song, a great, simple chant arising as if from thousands of voices in praise of the creator. Day and night its unvarying repetition continued, to the point of becoming maddening.

Yunshin, we learned, is the Ashaninca word for water spirit, but then the Maestro said he didn't know if there was one specifically for the half-human, half-fish we call mermaids, or *sirenas* as they are known in Spanish.

"There are many kinds of spirits of water," he said. "The sirena and *yacuruna,* the women and men of the waters. And there are other beings that have great power, such as the boa of the water, the yacumama."

The yacumama, he told us, is thirty to forty feet long, with bones of marble and multihued skin that flashes in the light. They live mainly in the lakes and in the renacales, but they transform themselves and go walking about from one place to another. They are spirits as well as animals: the sirena, the princess, and the doctor.

Juan went on to name other beings that live in the water, such as dragons, dolphins, and sea horses, as well as other potent creatures, such as the *anguila* who maintains an electric current within its body, and whose fat is very effective in treating certain diseases.

"Then there is the Sumiruna, who is the chief of all the spirits of the water and a great doctor. He is the master of all three realms: jungle, water, and sky. Less accomplished than the Sumiruna, there are two other kinds of shamans. The first is the *banco muraya,* who is the master of the plants and animals upon the land. The animal that accompanies him is the *banco puma,* the spotted jaguar who lives in the jungle. The other is the *sumi muraya,* the master of the underwater realms. He is accompanied by the *yana puma,* the black panther, who lives in the waters."

This distinction between shamans and their jaguar allies was news to us, and I scrambled to take notes.

"The culture below the water is very ancient and refined; all are kings and queens," he continued. "The kings are dragons, the queens are diamondlike, like the Sumiruna, no? As the lords of nature, they dwell in golden palaces. It's very beautiful, because they are the doctors, the princesses, and the seamstresses of the water. The sirenas also send messages when they sing—their song is very sad and can move anyone. So when they want to enchant someone, they come forth and sing. You can hear them, but it has to be in a moment of deep silence and you are left deeply moved."

I asked Juan if he had heard of Odysseus and his encounter with the sirens, and he shook his head no, so I related Homer's tale to him. I then commented that illustrations of the sirens depicted them surrounded by the skeletons of mariners unfortunate enough to have become addicted to their song.

"This is why tobacco is so important, as the director of plants and spirits," he commented. "The spirits of the water cannot take tobacco. It's too potent for them. I always take my mapachos with me when I travel. Whenever I travel by canoe, I give a soplada to the water for protection."

Images of the sailor, pipe clenched in teeth, came to us. Perhaps the old salts knew more than they had let on.

"But the sirens here seem to be different," I offered. "They seem more benevolent in nature."

The Maestro paused. "No, they're not," he stated flatly, and I remembered the story he had told us about his sister that now lives in the waters:

Florinda was stolen when she was very young. She was a very playful girl, and one day she was swimming with my brothers and one of my brothers realized something was happening to her. She was in the middle of the water, and something had seized her by the waist. Then there was only a single little hand, waving, as if my sister wanted to say good-bye, no? They already knew there was a sirena in the waters because they had seen it at a distance, and now it had taken her.

"It wasn't a yacumama, Maestro? A boa?"

No, it wasn't a boa. It was a person that lives in the waters called a sirena. Bueno, that's the way my sister disappeared. I didn't know anything about her for many years. I was very worried when I heard the news, and I returned home to Pucallpa to study what had really happened, because I had heard that eight days after drowning, the spirit walks about in its previous habitation. But I was there in my house for eight days and nothing happened. Not a sound. Not a step. Nothing.

So I left again, and many years passed. Then suddenly I was able to talk with my sister. She appeared and told me, "Bueno, I'm doing fine. Tranquilo. I don't live in this world anymore, but belong to the other." She hadn't died at all, although with the years she passed in the water her body wasn't the same anymore. She had married a yacuruna, one of the men of the water, and transformed into a princesa, a sirena. Now she is a curandera of the waters.

So from that time on I had the ability to consult with her, because among the many sicknesses that spring up on earth are those we call the sicknesses of the water, for which she knows many remedies. Sometimes these diseases attack a person when they don't know any better, for example, and start throwing stones in the waters of lakes, and the waters resent the blows and send a negative force. Or sometimes when people scuba dive without protection a spirit takes part of their soul.

I sometimes think it was our destiny to be this way, her as a curandera in the water, and me as a curandero on the land. In this way we can transmit our knowledge to each other.

It was only much later that I learned the fuller implications of Juan's narrative, both in terms of his status and the sharply divided nature of the underwater realm in Amazonian shamanism.

As reflected in Juan's narrative, the underwater realm is a two-edged sword: the place where, according to anthropologist Luis Eduardo Luna, "powerful shamans enjoy perfect affinal relations with their mermaid or mermen consorts in affluent cities is contrasted with the socially destructive acts of water spirits in abducting the weak and luring the strong into life-threatening dangers."[2] Intriguingly, Luna's study of four shamans in the Iquitos region of Peru offers an overview of this underwater realm closely paralleling Juan's vision:

> *In the basic cosmovision of the area . . . there are two parallel worlds, the world of the earth and the world of the water. The world of the water seems to be especially important. It is the home of the yacuruna and the sirenas (mermaids), who at times adopt human bodies and come out of the water, quite often for the purpose of copulating with humans or of stealing a partner to be taken to their underwater world. The yacuruna are very often associated and even identified with the bufeos (freshwater dolphins, considered malignant beings) and the mermaids with ana-condas (water boas). All four informants have an enormous repertoire of stories telling about one or another episode in which a woman or man was stolen and taken into the water, or about women who became boas during the night, thus revealing their true identity.[3]*

Additionally, according to the work of anthropologist Françoise Barbira Freedman (whose informants did not possess Juan's distinction between the sumi muraya and the banco muraya), "the highest *vegetalista* shamanic status" is the "*banco muraya,* shaman-diviner who has gained access to the underwater connections in the cosmos."[4]

Juan's connection with his abducted sister in the underwater realm, along with the fact that one of his main animal allies is a banco puma (who sits guard at the door to his maloca during ceremonies at Mayan-tuyacu), suggests that he has attained a high vegetalista status.

On the surface, our diet was as uneventful as hibernation. While the *plátano,* or green plantain, like a single, glowing ember, burned solo in our bellies, our bodies daily shrank like Incan mummies. Muscles cinched up tight from lack of salt. Stomachs became taut as drums. My nose pro-truded like a beak, and my mouth hinted of the grin of a skull. Susana had the face of a porcelain doll. I began feeling the bones of sacrum and spine crunching against the stone of the river whenever I went to sit by the stream.

Each day we watched the life of the jungle. The ducklings paddled around below us, sometimes raiding the kitchen for food scraps. Two brown squirrels with bushy tails that stood straight up like pine trees, and big, stocky bodies, more like badgers than the lean, ferretlike squirrels of the north, fished around the hot spring just down the way. We heard the cackling of monkeys, but we only occasionally saw them hanging from the limbs of trees extending out over the river. And I saw a wild pig—a humble character, bowed and light-footed, who disappeared with a ruckus into the trees. Long, whiplike snakes hissed warnings at us when we walked down the canyon.

One morning a tiny and extremely venomous cascabel lay curled up on the steps to the kitchen, unperturbed by the passing bare feet of myself and our aide, Brunswick. Susana, returning from her bath, discerned its deadly noose among the leaves and we trapped it, only to release it later at a distance from the camp.

The moon was our streetlight, and when the spirits were out dry lightning came down in huge, silent bursts, illuminating the river canyon like flashes of gunpowder.

In our weekly outings to the center to drink ayahuasca with the Maestro, the patients seemed engaged in frenetic activity, agitated with unnecessary bursts of indiscreet energy. As dictated by the rules of the diet, we touched no one and we talked little, and we were always relieved to depart and return to the primitive tambos that had become our homes.

But just below the surface, dreams of all species roiled.

With our external lights nearly doused, our inner lights flared.

The deep sonorous chant that accompanied Susana everywhere in the jungle grew more and more insistent. The pressure built until she finally thought, "Maybe I just need to sit down and try singing along." Taking out her pen and notebook, she began transcribing all the praise she could hear arising from the jungle to the elements and animals and plants and insects. As the pages and pages of verses accumulated, she took out her tape recorder and began to practice singing them. The next morning, she awoke to find the sound of the chant no longer ringing in her mind.

In the first days, I continued putting out Tigrilla's food bowls, leaving an offering in them for her spirit, unable to let go of her. Then one night I dreamed of returning home to the United States. Sitting in the airport waiting to board, I saw something struggling inside my carry-on bag. Mystified, I opened it and Tigrilla leaped out into my lap. I exclaimed, "You amazing cat! How did you manage to put yourself in there?" But then as she wound herself around me, I saw the empty sockets that were her eyes.

I never put out her food bowls again.

The fact is that the sudden death of Tigrilla, compounded with the intensity of months of internal journeying, had left me exhausted. At this stage of my pilgrimage, I had lived long outside the protective sphere of my own country, survived supernatural attacks, desperately sought allies through the most mysterious and dangerous world I had ever wandered in, and crossed thresholds I had never imagined existed.

There were times my body ached for the familiar: the granite and pine trees of the Sierra Nevada, motes of pollen lazily drifting in shafts of golden sunshine, manzanita and madrone, the creak of old wood in a dry summer, and bear roaming the forest—a world my animal nature recognized and knew. Like a deer caught in headlights, I had been in fight-or-flight reactions to oncoming dangers for too long. It was becoming a habit I needed to break.

The jungle concurred.

Previously, in sessions of ayahuasca I had seen the spirit of tobacco as a brilliant darting white light, swift as a hummingbird, coming to help me cleanse and set boundaries within myself. Now as I settled into dieting the root of the plant, I began to dream of tobacco in the simultaneous guise of my childhood best friend, Gordon, and as a tobacconist.

Dressed in a dapper blue sports jacket with a yachting insignia on its breast, he had first offered to sell me very expensive imported cigarettes. I declined, reacting from the guarded stance of poverty that had blighted my youth, stating I preferred my simple mapachos. The spirit diagnosed this: I was "suffering from internal poverty."

In the next dream I was a street kid again, caught back in cycles of homelessness. Finding myself in Gordon's house, I was conscious of the fineness of the wood, deeply oiled and rich, of the room I entered. It felt like I was in the heart of a tree. There, in finely carved blocks of wood, was spelled out a message of welcome to me and beneath it was a document with a pen beside it. Picking up the paper, I discovered it was a rental contract, offering me very generous terms to move into the house. I was deeply touched by the ceremonious formality of the invitation—there was no trace of charity to the poor in it. I awoke thinking, *Only Gordon had the power to invite me off the streets into his family home.*

In the roots of the plant the house of tobacco was nestled in, I felt the agitated, wandering spirit of my street days settling, finding rest and nourishment. Closure in the process begun months earlier in the purges at Takiwasi, which had seemed to tear me open without remedy.

Likewise, as the vital force of the plants penetrated our systems, Susana experienced the reawakening of symptoms long repressed.

One afternoon she turned to me and said, "Bito, I'm really scared."

She related how she had felt a thing like a dart enter her eye the day before, which in her rarified state she intuited was not an insect but a virus. Her eye was still in pain, and the symptoms were the same as the childhood corneal herpes that had nearly left her blind in one eye.

The herpes still flared up occasionally, and it meant she needed medicine to repress the attack immediately—a medicine prescribed in a specific clinic in Chile. If we played around with time, the herpes could damage her eye and leave her disabled. The disease appeared acute. We began calculating how quickly we could emerge from the jungle and get her to Santiago, if we left first thing in the morning.

Then in consultation with Juan, he told us the flare-up was normal in the process of dieting. Plants *"sacan el mal,"* he assured us, take the disease lingering in the body out. What felt like a renewed attack on her eye was actually the herpes departing her system for good. Although this was contrary to our received wisdom, and the outcome would be very costly if Juan proved incorrect, we chose to trust him, meanwhile carefully monitoring the progress of the pain in her eye.

That evening, under the catalyzing effects of ayahuasca, the disease was extracted, drawn out through all the links in its chain of causation.

As the Maestro sang at the height of the ceremony, our spirit cat came to Susana in her state of mareación and began licking her eye, comforting her. As she got in touch with the powerful loyalty of Tigrilla, a portion of her deep memory stirred, and she began reconnecting with the loyalty she had felt to her mother as a very young girl just before the first onset of her herpes symptoms. Depressed and abandoned in a bad marriage, her mother had demonstrated the misery of life so strongly that Susana preferred to blind herself rather than see, out of loyalty, through her mother's eyes. As she cried and cried during the ceremony, Tigrilla stayed with her, licking her eye. Gradually the pain began to go down, as the entire etiology of the disease emerged into consciousness.

Within a couple of days, Susana's symptoms passed away entirely. Her recovery was evident, even to those who knew nothing about the dangerous flare-up. Out walking, she encountered Ivan, a visitor to the center from Canada out hunting seeds and feathers on the forest floor. His first comment on seeing her was, "Your eyes are brighter and rounder than I've ever seen them!"

With this event I realized that I had witnessed the workings of one of the most ancient principles of medicine, what the earliest Greek Hippocratic texts called coction.

In coction the sick, raw organism is "cooked" so that the "crude sediment" of disease floats to the surface and is refined away. The Hippocratic physician did not interrupt disease by counteracting and repressing it.[5] He could only stimulate or deflect it, observing and interpreting the character of the pathology and interceding at the moment of crisis with a medicine sympathetic to the disease (i.e., healing) process. In this original form of medicine, at the right moment a good doctor intensifies the disease, playing the keynote that musters the vital force and triggers its full flux, allowing it to pass entirely from the organism. Otherwise, according to Théophile Bordeu, one of the fathers of hormonal medicine, "quelling the symptoms at crisis insured a history of chronic disease."[6]

Bordeu also "believed that mineral springs were powerfully medicinal because they could transform chronic diseases back into acute ones through inciting coction."[7] In the true spirit of vegetalismo, he also "praised the cure-all theriaca, which was made up of all the leftover medicines from an apothecary's shop at the end of the day. He saw it, like mineral waters, as peppy and stimulating, awaking the vital force from its languor and from its dwelling in melancholy and suppressed anger."[8]

As in the work of Juan, the Hippocratic physician had to choose medicines of the right intensity and type: "too early a response might have retarded the accumulating current, and too strong a dose might have snapped the vital force and killed the patient."[9] As Juan put it, the shaman must know when to fire and have sufficient energy to catalyze and carry through the healing.

In the last days of the diet, we went transparent and dreamed the jungle, or it dreamed us. Coherence of narrative once again vanished. Among the vivid, inexplicable images that remain, there is one that captures the mystery of our communion with the spirits of the plants:

It is of one night in ceremony, of myself seated before the Maestro as he sang the icaro of the shihuahuaco over me, feeling the vibrations of his voice spreading like roots in my belly, weaving harmonic patterns in my psyche, reknitting places the jarring concussions of hard travel had left in my internal landscape. Then visions of trees, endless trees, kaleidoscopic, crowding upon me. Susana, glancing over at the Maestro's seat, saw not my human form but a shihuahuaco tree spreading its limbs before him, my head transformed into the great, rustling canopy of the stately tree, my thoughts birds singing in the sheltering, green branches. Then when the Maestro blew smoke over me, she felt it simultaneously upon her own face, connected as we now were within the spirit of the tree.

I had become the green man, my body empty of anything inside but trees.

At the end of thirty days, we broke the diet with a small ritual and ate a meal different from the one I had been fantasizing about for a month: an anticlimactic, watery soup of chicken and vegetables. I braved a papaya, spooning its rubbery slivers into my hollow mouth. For dessert, we sprinkled pinches of salt onto our tongues.

That evening in ceremony, Juan called us to his seat. Leaning forward in the darkness, he quietly explained that he was about to bestow *arkana* on us. We had heard this word before, from don Martín the trickster, and we knew the word came from the Quechua *arkarta*—defense. We also had a general idea of its tradition in Amazonian medicine, but this was the first time we had heard the Maestro speak of it.

"This arkana icaro is given to persons who have done long diets, and all of them have gone well. Then the master makes an evaluation of their comportment, because these arkana are crowns that are given as a gift. They are not erasable and stay until one's dying day. In this case, the arkana belong to you because you have done good work and have dieted well. The spirits came and we conversed and I told them, 'These are people who should receive the arkana. They deserve it for their defense their whole life long.'

"The arkana are composed first of a pair of shoes made of steel, so a person can walk wherever he desires and nothing negative can enter through his feet. Then he carries two swords on both sides of his belt in sheaths. Continuing up the body, in both hands he holds a sword. Finally, he wears a helmet [Juan used the word *sombrero*] of steel to protect the head.

"The word *arkana* is the circle of medicine that includes all the instruments received during your diet, to receive the arkana of protection within the body. The swords are of steel so everything shines within the person in opposition to evil spirits. There are very black spirits that we curanderos have to protect ourselves from when studying how to heal and serve humanity.

"This icaro is very rarely heard in other places. It isn't practiced in the medicine of other curanderos. Maybe they have other types of arkana, but this is an arkana that comes from long, long ago that my master transmitted to me and that I am transmitting to my followers in the art of traditional medicine. I give this icaro to very few people. I have to very much desire to give it," he concluded.

I felt a surge of anticipation and relief arise in me. We had dieted well and he had decided we merited the gift.

Returning to my seat, I listened to him sing for Susana. Then Juan called me forward and as he sang I felt his voice inscribing the images of armature upon me, flowing and staccato, like the tip of a painter's brush. After drinking a second cup of ayahuasca, I returned to my seat.

Like a dark wave, the ayahuasca penetrated my system. I suddenly felt adrift—badly adrift, and filled with foreboding. Juan sat silently, having finished the individual healings. Navigating my way to his seat, I asked him, nearly begged him, to sing for me.

The Maestro sat silently for a long time. Then he began the very long icaro enumerating all the plants and calling their spirits, the one he called "the parade" when he was in a joking mood. In a moment, the mareación hit with consciousness-fragmenting power, and as the plants passed by, his voice transformed in timbre, its resonance deepening and widening. I heard Yahweh, the Ancient of Days, giving the earth to Adam and Eve.

The *first* voice, the voice in the garden, the voice of Yahweh. A song heard long ago in the human species' cradle . . .

Juan stood and phosphorus blazed above me. *Uhhhhh, just a moment here,* I managed to reason as he blew smoke and perfume on me. *I heard the voice of Yahweh, sure as any prophet in old Israel. But that icaro invoked the power of nature. If I'm really regressed back to the origins of mind, then this could be empirical evidence that the* voice *our ancestors heard in the garden came from the power of the garden* itself, *not some deity set above and beyond it. As the Maestro told me, Christ is incarnate in the plants. . . .*

Nursing my mapacho before the Maestro, contemplating this sudden reversal in my metaphysics, the velocity of my consciousness began to wheel out of control. The white figure of Brunswick began to appear and disappear in different sections of the maloca, as if he were moving at the speed of light. The Maestro still sat in front of me, but with the solidity of a flickering candle. The interstices of time and space opened. It was either that or my awareness was accelerating to such a degree that the normal movie projector processing speed of consciousness appeared for what it was: full of holes.

And at such speeds, what was my "I"? Prostrate before the Maestro, I dreamed of Christ rising from his tomb in the fifteenth-century fresco in the church of the Knights of Santiago in Galicia, before which I had stood as a pilgrim to Santiago years before. The light of Christ's wounds burst upon me like suns, cleansing me.

But the speed was still too much.

"I am . . . I am . . . I am . . . ," I chanted, reaching for identity, for ancient memory. "I am one with the light, with the saviors of deep consciousness, with the endless source of being. I die and am reborn, but I am never separate, never alone. I and the father are one."

I could settle, surely I could settle. I could ride this one out. . . .

Suddenly there was a mob of spirits, an endless series of obstacles intruding themselves before the light. *What is this dark shape inside me?* I wondered. Lean as trees, we had broken our month-long diet that morning with a chicken soup, and I saw the consciousness of the bewildered chicken I had eaten inside me. There it was, wondering what in the world to do with itself. . . .

The ancient, uncompromising traditions of fasting came to me, such as the *enduras* to death of the medieval Cathar, who in daily life abstained from meat to avoid taking the duller consciousness of animals into them. *I've fasted myself into a rare condition indeed,* I thought, as I prayed for the good rebirth of the chicken I was carrying in my stomach.

The Ancient of Days was not the only voice I was to reckon with that evening.

The Adversary was also perfectly recognizable when it struck. Mara, the dragon, Satan, the Matrix, whatever god or metaphysical construct we employ to depict the Enemy, the devourer of consciousness—he made his move as I fragmented beyond the hopelessly plodding speed of thought. *His* was the voice of damnation, addressing my *knowing* I was hopelessly lost, a knowledge that reached beyond the perimeters of this life into the network of eternity—ineluctable and inscribed into the foundations of my being.

Bleating in terror, my habitual self panicked and immediately surrendered before the onslaught of childhood nightmare. Its need for self-preservation, for a velocity of consciousness in which it could recognize its own image, was now as dangerous as the Adversary.

The memory of Juan's gift came to me, and I drew my sword. Scrambling at ever-increasing velocities of flashing dream, my survival in the realm of spirit lay in moving in accord with its reality as I thrust and fought and struggled free again and again. Staying barely one step ahead of the enemy, I managed a cut with my blade. A clean slice to my own brain, just above the forehead, on the right side of the frontal lobe, performed with surgical accuracy.

The operation achieved, a deadly repetition set in, the thrashing tail of the dying dragon. Burying my head in Susana's lap, I sought relief from the coils of images winding around my psyche and pulling me into oblivion. She gently shook a shacapa of basil over my head and chatted with the Maestro. I heard her comment from somewhere in my dream, "He's dieted so long, his head is as tiny as a chicken's."

It was a night for chickens. I vomited into her lap.

She laughed and cleaned it up.

The night wore on. Scenes of jail and torture kept claiming me and dragging me down. Information about how my soul was lost, how I was a loner, forever cut off from the love of others, kept engulfing me. I began to fear I was trapped in the warped velocities of spirit forever. My soul would never know rest again.

Burrowing into Susana, I told her how much I loved her, how she was my light.

"God, when you look at me with those eyes you scare me!" she laughed.

The blazing eyes of the trapped man, the sociopath loner. As much as I fought him, he kept surfacing. I *was* him.

Finally I could fight no longer. My energy was flagging. Softened, looking into Susana's eyes as the eyes of Santa María herself, I told her I had to let go and die. Stroking my hair, she told me it was okay. I could die. I gave up. What would be in eternity would be. I could fight no more.

Susana began walking me around the maloca like a drunk. Again I fell vomiting to the floor, again she picked me up and walked me. Finally, my body began showing signs of being mine again.

Then the consolation came. The good things of the earth returned to me one by one. Clutching Susana's knees, I put my forehead on them and said, "My love, I've done it. I've died and returned again."

"Welcome to the new world," she replied.

It was like my eyelids had been torn off. Each step, breath, word with Susana was infinitely precious: a dance.

Alone on the trail, I see a single star penetrating through the canopy of glowering rain clouds: a diamond light seeing me, entering me. My body adjusts itself into the star-receiving yoga posture. Opening my arms and arching my back to the sky, I feel the consciousness of the star brushing over me. It retreats behind the clouds when Susana comes down the path and I point up to the sky. The moment of supernal connection has passed, and a living star is no spectacle.

How extraordinarily limited is the conceptual habitat of Western science, I think, fallen under the spell of two English "empiricists" who would forbid humanity to perceive purpose and higher orders of intelligence in nature. (A case in point being the dull droning in the classrooms and textbooks about how the speed of light is 186,000 miles a second and therefore what we see in the sky are images of stars and galaxies transmitted from times of inconceivable antiquity. A portrait gallery of stars already long burnt out.)

The first of these empiricists was William of Ockham, a fourteenth-century English friar and logician who introduced a tenet to medieval philosophy known subsequently as Occam's razor. It still holds invisible, and tyrannical, sway over our minds: *entia non sunt multiplicanda praeter necessitatem,* which translates awkwardly to: "entities should not be multiplied beyond necessity." In other words, the simplest, most economical explanation is preferable to a complicated, fancy one. We can all embrace this, yet as Einstein commented, "Everything should be as simple as it can be, but not simpler." When a purely metaphysical tenet converts into unconscious dogma that restricts freedom of thought, we have a problem.

For example, one of the guiding principles of the study of animal behavior, Morgan's canon, restates Ockham's razor in this way, "In no case may we interpret an action as the outcome of the exercise of a higher psychical faculty, if it can be interpreted as the outcome of the exercise of one which stands lower in the psychological scale."[10] This, of course, is pure prejudice, yet, "For decades, psychologists, biologists, linguists, and philosophers used Morgan's canon to deny the mental experiences of animals."[11] How then would these psychologists and animal researchers approach Tigrilla's role in healing the outbreak of herpes in Susana's eye? What is the simplest and most obvious explanation—that the spirit of our cat came to her aid—must go through a tortuous process of reinterpretation and denial to conclude it was all a subjective experience, mostly hallucination, which can be safely dismissed as auto-suggestion because it does not fit in with the rationalist tenets of modern science, never mind the pesky empirical evidence.

The second empiricist was Francis Bacon, best known for his dictum, "knowledge is power." According to philosopher Louis Dupré, Bacon's call for "unlimited control over nature rested on the assumption that nature possessed no purpose of its own. Well before mechanistic philosophy, he eliminated final causality from scientific investigation, comparing it to a consecrated virgin who bears no offspring. His opposition to teleological interpretations . . . placed the entire responsibility for conveying meaning and purpose to the world entirely on the human person, the only creature endowed with purposiveness."[12]

The final cause, as formulated by Aristotle, is the purpose, or the inherent intelligence of a thing or event. In other words, what is something *for* in and of itself? What is its *inherent* value beyond human utility, or even human existence? Where does it fit in the greater intelligence of a living cosmos? In Bacon's pragmatism, by eliminating purpose from the universe, the integration of humanity with nature is lost, and "the mastery of nature becomes its own end."[13]

As a consequence, modern science has lost interest in *what* the universe is, and it dismisses inquiries into final causes as unanswerable or belonging to metaphysical speculation. All that matters in a dead, mechanistic universe is how we can control it. As Richard Tarnas asks,

> *Is it not an extraordinary act of human hubris—literally, a hubris of cosmic proportions—to assume that the exclusive source of* all meaning and purpose *in the universe is ultimately centered in the human mind, which is therefore absolutely unique and special and in this sense superior to the entire cosmos? To base our entire world view on the a priori principle that whenever human beings perceive any patterns of psychological or spiritual significance in the nonhuman world, any signs of interiority and mind, any suggestion of purposefully coherent order and intelligible meaning, these must be understood as no more than human constructions and projections, as ultimately rooted in the human mind and never in the world? And that is why, Virginia, the stars must be dead, and there be no intelligence in the universe—no matter what the evidence of our senses tells us to the contrary.*[14]

Yet the naked eye sees what equations and telescopes cannot: at higher speeds of apprehension light emerges as sentient and simultaneously existing throughout the scape of time.

After saying good night to each other a thousand times, Susana was gone, a figure of white vanishing into the night. I was alone with my amplified faculties of soul. Taking my pipe, I sat by the river, smoking until morning. Then I slept with a closing of eyes like sunshine reflecting on water and awoke with no sense of time having passed. I was still amplified.

I found the Maestro with Susana and Henarte down in the Cocina para Medicina. The ayahuasca we had been preparing was in its final stages, the sacks of vine and leaf we had ritually prepared, stacked, and covered with water in vat after vat reduced down to thick caramel syrup after days of steaming over a blazing hot fire.

Taking the final vestiges of the process, we filtered it through an old, clean T-shirt, and then squeezing the bag like a tit, we milked the last possible amount of syrup out. As we labored around the pot, a lightning storm erupted: a gathering of the spirits of the valley of Mayantuyacu, imbuing themselves into the potion in their elemental forms.

Oh god, I thought as the atmosphere reared violently, explosions close at hand, flashes striking the eyes in broad daylight. *This is out of Macbeth. Enough mareación.*

"Just a little more work," I heard a woman's voice saying to me. "Just the briefest of travails, and it will be done."

That evening's storm lit up the deluged landscape with the brilliance of a noonday sun, revealing swollen rivers and sodden jungle as its atmosphere-rending thunder exploded in our faces like cannon. Leaning on the railing beneath the maloca's thatched roof, we passed the evening watching the structures built along the streams being carried away like so many leaves.

A subdued morning came. Pent up inside my cabin at the mercy of nibbling insects, I sought out Susana and found her lying in a hammock in the maloca, as irritable as me. Trudging back up to my cabin, I pulled on my rubber boots, picked up my machete, and headed for the jungle. It was a good day for a farewell walk through the landscape we were soon to depart, not to mention for hunting the brilliant little red and black seeds called *wayruro* used in the *artesanía* of the region.

Hiking up out of the valley, I passed the last banana plants and outlying tambos and entered the forest canopy. Streams were still running high, and the massive, soaked roots of the renacales and other trees twisted like brilliant-hued snakes through the soil. The air was washed clean of biting insects, and everywhere improvised streams and springs bubbled, balancing out the fresh weight of water in the earth. Keeping an eye out for snakes, I headed off on an unknown trail, before coming upon strange, thorn-studded trees and giant twisting vines thick as the cables of a suspension bridge. Large, raucous black birds fringed with brilliant plumage stayed one tree ahead of me. A grove stank of recent monkey habitation.

Reflecting on my months in Mayantuyacu, I felt how my machete had become second nature in my hand, and how my reverent awe for the jungle had vanished. Now, after the diet, I could truly say that I had come to love the plants—to feel their root systems running through me, their moisture washing me clean. The hair on the crown of my head transformed into leaves and my thoughts into singing birds like the shihuahuaco tree. Basically I had become an ent dieting and drinking its bark. It was good beyond my deepest hopes in coming to this foreign land and literally physically opening myself up to it.

Juan had told us that concealed within the shihuahuaco tree was a stone, brilliant like a diamond, that gives power to anyone who possesses it, but you must be very fast to see it and grab it, because when the tree is cut down the stone very quickly vanishes into the air. I wondered why anyone would want to take the magic of the shihuahuaco by force. How could anyone appreciate the extraordinary gifts of the tree taking root and growing inside by stealing its virtue?

The bright red wayruro were lying scattered about, half-nestled into the soil. Content like a little boy gathering Easter eggs, I collected the exposed ones and rooted about with my machete for others concealed in the duff. Ending up with a generous handful of the seeds the locals consider to be good luck, I left a single one lying in the path by way of thanks and continued on.

A tiny homestead was reached at the confluence of a number of streams, whose brown waters flowed high and smooth like polished marble through the dense green. Leaping the exposed stone across the river, I reached the farther shore and walked through the sandy soil among banana, yucca, and pepper plants, climbing over the smooth trunks of fallen trees. I had been to this locale before by a different route, and there never seemed to be anyone there, yet the farm was always immaculate. Two large ducks, a brown one and a white one, approached proprietarily, wagging their tail feathers and accompanying me about.

The homestead consisted of two main structures: one was a large, covered kitchen area with a huge rectangular hearth made of split logs. Opposite stood a long, sturdy table of dark wood, with metal plates neatly stacked in a rack and various bottles and implements sitting and hanging about. In the middle of a floor carefully strewn with the tough husks of seeds stood a large, upright grinding bowl, carved like a canoe out of a single section of log, with a huge pestle—two-headed like a paddle—hanging above it.

The air circulated easily. There was not a scrap of refuse to be seen.

The opposite structure, the sleeping and living quarters, had a thatched roof secured with the artistry of a basket weaver. The floor consisted of finely planed halved logs. Hammocks and buckets were suspended from above. I sat on the edge of it, dangling my legs and smoking a mapacho.

A shirt, hung from a rafter, clearly displayed the label GAP.

Sitting there in contemplation, I felt that simple wonder of things well made by hand, something in the spirit of the people as self-sufficient as the trees. I walked over to the ducks' house. Five extra large eggs in a wooden box.

Following the river downstream, the water flowed imperceptibly through silent canyons, the forest becoming more pristine and untouched with every step. *Is this paradise or what?* I thought placidly.

Floating spots danced like motes before my eyes. Fire erupted in different parts of my body and quicker than you can say the word "wasps," I was crashing through the trees, running toward a waterfall. Arriving, I plunged my arm into the water and counted four stings on it and on my back.

Chastened, I followed the swollen river back to Mayantuyacu, going in waist deep in the sections where the banks had disappeared. With water sloshing in my boots, I encountered Brunswick coming down the trail, armed to the hilt: rifle on shoulder, machete in hand, hunting knife hanging from leather sheath on his belt. I showed him my rapidly swelling right hand.

"The jungle's saying good-bye to you," he said, laughing.

Susana was in considerably better spirits when I arrived.

"Bito, I have incredible news," she said. "Carolina just wrote. They finished the medical exams and the tumor is gone! And she has no more diabetes!"

We looked at each other a stunned moment.

"Hallelujah!" I exclaimed, in the face of a patent miracle.

I found the Maestro down by the river in the Cocina para Medicina, wearing his Yoda hat and chopping wood for a new batch of ayahuasca he was brewing. He was beaming.

"Maestro, I want to congratulate you on the cure of Carolina. You are a Maestro indeed."

"Ya, Rober," he said, resting his axe and sitting down on a log. He was grinning like a little boy again, but this time it was obvious his magic trick had taken even him by surprise. We sat savoring the good news. My right hand was so swollen it looked like the Pillsbury Doughboy's.

Changing the subject, I narrated the events of the ceremony, of entering into velocities beyond my ability to navigate and the attack of the Adversary. "When it attacked I remembered the arkana you gave me and drew my sword to fight it."

"Yes, that's what arkana is for."

"Well, actually I spent most of my time running for my life. It was a dragon, after all. . . ."

"Then you did a spiritual operation."

"Yes . . . Maestro, I died. When I let go of the battle, when I surrendered, I faced the possibility that I was going to be extinguished. The end of the road, the snuffing out of my spirit for eternity. The dragon and I had to go down together."

"And you see how life continues. . . ."

"I have never felt such fear before."

"When you have fear, just say, *Ya, yo soy otorongo!*" he said, waving his hand to dismiss a hoard of attacking demons and spirits. Enough, I'm a jaguar!

"Ino Moxo, the black panther, was very powerful last night."

"Ya, Rober."

"I saw I am Ino Moxo."

"Yes, you are an otorongo."

"I actually am," I said slowly. It was, after all, simple arithmetic. "Maestro, how is this possible?"

"When you first drink the plant, you begin to transform. As you continue your transformation into the otorongo, you will understand more and more."

"Hmmm. What does God have to say about this? Are we supposed to be passing over the boundaries of form?"

"God says use the plants to transform," Juan intoned, nodding his head.

"And what about . . . demons? *Los diablitos?*" I said, using his term for the little diabolic forces that can easily penetrate the body when it is weak or toxic and take up residence in it.

"They are part of the other side. We work with the good, the force of creation."

I was able to accept the idea that I was becoming an otorongo. Somehow the fact that I was not inherently an otorongo, but rather was transforming into one through the properties of the plant, seemed an acceptable proposition.

On the other hand, our impending return to the human world appeared fraught with difficulty. I had always felt an exile within my own culture, and I had always tasted the metallic tinge of the prison system on my tongue. But now, I reflected sitting with Juan by the boiling river, I was more familiar with the root systems and overspreading branches of a shihuahuaco tree than the labyrinthine bureaucracies of the world economy.

Thinking of the battles raging just outside the borders of Mayantuyacu, I asked him, "Maestro, when are things finally going to begin to change for the better?"

"Ah, we have much work to do before then. It is going to get very hard. The first thing we have to do is invite all the presidents of the world to a *purga*," he concluded, laughing.

9 THE HOLY TREE

*The Voice spoke like someone weeping,
and it said: "Look there upon your
nation." And when I looked down, the
people were all changed back to human,
and they were thin, their faces sharp, for
they were starving. Their ponies were
only hide and bones, and the holy tree
was gone.*

BLACK ELK

Even as we prepared to leave the Shangri-la of Mayantuyacu to reenter the outside world, it came banging at
the gates.

During our immersion in the jungle, we had
received little outside news. Word filtered in about
another election in the United States redolent of fraud,
of a terrible wave that had consumed the coast of Asia,
but perhaps the most significant news we heard came
from the mouth of Juan himself. "There's not enough
rain," he commented one evening, looking up at the sky
ruefully. "Normally at this time of year, there is much
more rain."

Global warming.

We also didn't need any newspaper headlines to see the oil pipelines running across the path leading into Mayantuyacu, or to interpret the occasional helicopters that came pounding across the sky. *"Petroleros,"* said Juan. Petroleum companies.

Mayantuyacu, like countless other regions of the Amazon, is presently under siege. As we chafe watching the meters click on our gasoline pumps to the tempo of soaring oil company profits, native peoples are paying with their health and lives throughout the Amazon. These crimes, committed by the oil companies, international banks, and collaborating politicians, are done in the same spirit of ruthless efficiency as the original conquistadors and Indian killers—and they are happening as you read this.

Upstream from the same Ucayali river that flows through Pucallpa, an invasion is occurring into native lands by oil companies. Entitled the Camisea Natural Gas Project, this move to extract natural gas and oil from the Urubamba basin in Peru—one of the most fragile and biodiverse regions of the Amazon—has already proved genocidal.*

A state reserve had been deliberately created by the government of Peru in 1990 to protect the vulnerable Nahua, Nanti, and Kirineri tribes from outside intrusion. Original contact with the peoples living in this region was made by Shell while conducting gas exploration in the mid 1980s. Forty-two percent of the Nahua people subsequently died from the diseases introduced by this contact.

These people are vulnerable for a reason. It is a well-known scientific fact that native peoples of the Americas do not have immunity to the diseases of Eurasia. As Jared Diamond states in his classic study *Guns, Germs, and Steel,* "Smallpox, measles, influenza, typhus, bubonic plague and other infectious diseases endemic in Europe played a decisive role in

---

*All of the information in this chapter on the history of the Camisea project and the environmental crimes of Texaco (now Chevron) in northern Ecuador is drawn, unless noted, from the website of Amazon Watch. Amazon Watch is one of the most effective grassroots environmental organizations presently working to defend the Amazon. They can be contacted at amazonwatch.org.

European conquests, by decimating many peoples on other continents."[1] In many cases, up to 90 percent of native tribes died as a result of these infectious diseases before a white man could even appear on the horizon.

It was statistically predictable, therefore, that Shell's incursion would result in massive death in the region. One wonders if the question ever arose in the minds of the executives at Shell, sitting in their plush skyscraper boardrooms, if such deaths were really necessary for the sake of progress.

To continue the saga: As I write this, a consortium of companies has mounted a full-scale invasion of the reserve, in violation of international laws such as ILO Convention 169 and the American Declaration on the Rights of Indigenous Peoples. One of these companies is Hunt Oil—a Dallas-based company with close ties to the Bush administration. Chief Executive Ray L. Hunt contributed to President Bush's presidential campaign and also sits on the board of Halliburton, the company formerly headed by Vice President Dick Cheney.

Another of the companies in this consortium, Pluspetrol, has a record of leaving behind devastation easily paralleling the human and environmental cost of the Exxon Valdez oil spill. In one of Peru's largest protected areas, the Pacaya-Samiria National Reserve, an oil spill by Pluspetrol has seriously affected the health of the Cocama-Cocamilla people, who suffered severe diarrhea, skin diseases, and malnutrition after their food and water supplies were contaminated by toxic pollution. In the northern Peruvian Amazon, Pluspetrol continues to pump oil wastes into local rivers, causing stomach ailments, cancer, and respiratory diseases among Achuar and Quichua communities.

As part of the Camisea invasion, employees of Veritas (ironically meaning "truth" in Latin), a contractor working for Pluspetrol, have forced additional contact, pressuring tribes to abandon their ancestral lands. Pluspetrol also facilitated the transportation of missionaries, by helicopter, to remote areas to contact isolated indigenous groups, in a fine illustration of Jared Diamond's definition of priests as those employed to "provide religious justification for wars of conquest."[2]

Fear of extinction has driven the Nahua to take the unprecedented step of publicly communicating, through local advocates, their rejection of all oil and gas operations within their lands:

In the past, Shell worked here and almost all of us died from the diseases. . . . We know that if another company comes here, our rivers and land will be destroyed. What will we eat when the rivers are dead and the animals have run away?[3]

As the fish and game stocks are depleted as a consequence of project construction, small children are already at risk from chronic malnutrition. As well, dozens of new cases of syphilis were reported by the health post in the indigenous community of Kirigueti. "Now there is such a combination of illnesses that we can't identify the illnesses that we get," stated one native of the region."[4]

In addition, Hunt Oil has acquired another oil concession adjacent to the Block 88 they are presently exploiting. The demands of indigenous organizations for a transparent, free, and informed consultation process regarding the opening of this additional territory were ignored, and nearly four million acres of rainforest now lie vulnerable to the effects of gas extraction.

Paradoxically, while disasters like Exxon Valdez continue to receive media scrutiny years after that event, a near total blackout of coverage exists for current catastrophes in the Amazon that dwarf the ecological consequences of the Alaskan oil spill. Is this because we have become habituated after five hundred years to the deaths of indigenous populations, just like the deaths of the buffalo and the wolf? Or is it just because we don't really want to know the dirty details of where that gasoline we just injected into our car came from?

A second grim example lies to the north in Ecuador. There, between 1964 and 1992, Texaco/Chevron operated a concession from the Ecuadorian government to extract oil in the northern jungle, and in a cold analysis of cost versus benefit, it saved four and a half billion dollars by not investing in reinjection equipment. In other words, oil extraction is analogous to sucking blood out of the earth, and the black gore that is not refined off must be injected back where it came from. This is the law in the United States and throughout most of the world. But in Ecuador, Texaco struck gold. According to William Langewiesche,

> *When Texaco signed the contract, [Ecuador] was not with a representative government, but with an incompetent military regime in a corrupt country . . . where the indigenous people were not even recognized as full citizens. Ecuador had practically no environmental regulations, no technical knowledge of oil operations, no scientific or public-health expertise, no governmental oversight capabilities—and no clue it even needed such things.*[5]

In a ruthless exploitation of this bonanza, Texaco dumped eighteen billion gallons of toxic waste, including more pure crude than was spilled in the Exxon Valdez disaster, into over a thousand open pits and into the rivers flowing over an area the size of Rhode Island. These were waters that six indigenous tribes drank and washed in and fished in.

Only five tribes of the original six now remain. Among those five an epidemiological study published in the prestigious *International Journal of Occupation and Environmental Health* found rates of cancer 130 percent above Ecuador's norm. Another study found ninety-one cases of child leukemia and rates of child cancer four times higher than the norm. Other peer-reviewed scientific studies have found elevated rates of oil-related health problems such as spontaneous miscarriages and genetic defects.

These waters, by the way, fall on *our* cities and *our* fields of waving grain.

In the open pits, some the size of Olympic swimming pools, where these wastes lie, 100 percent of the thirty-five inspected sites whose results have been reported in court demonstrate significant amounts of life-threatening toxins, some thousands of times above the maximum amounts permitted both by Ecuadorian and U.S. law. One site, Lago 2, contained total petroleum hydrocarbons (TPHs) in the soil at 325,000 parts per million—an astounding 3,250 times higher than permitted in California, Chevron's home state.

As in the case of perpetrators of war crimes, Texaco committed this act in full consciousness of the human and environmental suffering their policies would cause, prompting legal scholars to suggest that Chevron should be charged with genocide under international criminal law. In court, their main strategy is denial. According to Langewiesche, Chevron "denies that their soil and water samples are meaningful, denies that the methods the company used to extract oil in the past were substandard, denies that it contaminated the forest, denies that there is a link between the drinking water and high rates of cancer, leukemia, birth defects and skin disease . . . and, for added measure, denies that it bears responsibility for any environmental damage that might after all be found to exist."[6]

Sadly, the only shred of truth may lie in Chevron's claim that "Texaco always complied with Ecuadorean law."[7]

Thankfully, in the descending darkness of recent years as the government of Peru has sold off concessions to 70 percent of its territory, up from only 11 percent in 2004, there are bursts of light.

One came recently in what Dan Collyns in *The Guardian* called "by any measure a remarkable protest." According to the article:

More than 800 Achuar tribespeople from the borders of Peru and Ecuador, headed by their traditional leaders with their red and yellow feathered headdresses, arrived last month by the boatload in the twilight hours at four oil wells in the middle of the Amazonian rainforest.

Their faces streaked with paint and with some of them carrying hunting shotguns and ceremonial spears, they formed a peaceful blockade of Peru's largest oil facility. They stayed for nearly two weeks, shutting down power to most of the region's oil production and its road, airport, and river access.

It was a desperate attempt by the Achuar to get the Peruvian govern-

ment to take notice of their plight. For decades they had been saying that their land had been heavily polluted and their waters poisoned by oil exploration, but they had been consistently ignored.

The plan worked. The loss of millions of dollars in revenue and around 40,000 barrels of oil per day forced the government and Pluspetrol—Peru's largest oil and gas operator—to concede to most of the Achuar's demands, including reinjecting all the contaminated waste water back into the ground within two years, and building a new hospital with enough money to run a health service for ten years.

The victory was particularly sweet for the Achuar—who number around 8,000 in Peru's vast Amazon region of Loreto—because it was the first time in thirty-six years of oil exploration and extraction in their area that the state had intervened.[8]

These were the echoes of the terrible struggles we heard every time a helicopter pounded through the sky. Nor did we need news broadcasts to hear the terrible crash of trees falling around Mayantuyacu or simulcam technology to view them hauled out through the mud like great corpses.

Deforestation. The converting of the Amazon, the great moist lungs of the planet, into a vast grassland, the Serengeti of South America. Twenty percent of the oxygen you are breathing right now, and 50 percent of the rain that falls on the plains of Iowa to moisten our fields of grain, come from this wet ecosystem, and we are killing it as certainly as a smoker of manufactured cigarettes kills his own lungs.

We knew the grim figures: 17–18 percent of the jungle is already dead, another 20 percent is seriously degraded. Yet we continue to cut at the rate of seventy-five hundred square miles a year, or six soccer fields a minute. The Amazon has reached the tipping point. If the incursions go much deeper, according to scientists such as Thomas Lovejoy,[9] the system will begin to collapse upon itself and this will not be gradual. It will be exponential, accelerating so rapidly some of us may see the death of the greatest forest on the planet in our lifetime.

Back on the local front, it was Hermano, bitter with poverty and hypnotized by the visions of easy money, who opened a gate to "progress."

The owner of land adjacent to Mayantuyacu, Hermano scraped a living out of the soil with a little *chacra,* a small plantation of bananas, yucca, and papayas. He often came to visit us, a little man wearing a soiled baseball cap and trailing a friendly dog. Rambling in, he paid court to the Maestro, joined in the meals, and mingled with staff and patients, cracking jokes and resorting to Juan in hard times for small gifts of money or healings.

The Maestro welcomed him to ceremonies, and he had even led him in a traditional diet deep in the jungle, introducing him to the spirits of the plants that Hermano lived around every day. Juan also encouraged him to take advantage of the foreign visitors to Mayantuyacu by developing a cottage industry where he could sell his products, whether handicrafts or wasp honey, to the wealthy *extranjeros.* Hermano never exhibited much interest in that sort of work.

But taking Susana and I aside one day, he did offer us the skin of a young puma he had shot. We declined, saying we preferred to see them living. He took the point with a smile.

Then one morning Sandra received a radio message from Mayantuyacu. It was the Maestro, incoherent with tears. Finally, Brunswick got on the line and explained the situation. Word had just reached them that Hermano had sold the giant medicinal trees on his land to a timber company. The years of mentoring and support of the little campesino had been futile. Hermano had not only done this behind the back of his master, but he had not even offered Mayantuyacu the option to purchase the land in lieu of the timber company.

When the Maestro and Sandra went to speak with Hermano, it was a different man who emerged from the darkness of his corrugated tin–roofed house. His chest thrust forward, Hermano now strutted like a rooster. Reminding him of the gifts that the jungle had given him, Juan tried to call his errant disciple home.

"Ya, yo no soy ecologista!" Hermano declared, thumping his chest. "Enough! I'm not an ecologist!"

"But what is your land going to be worth without the trees?" they asked him. "The trees are your wealth, as well as the health of your land. Your land will die without them."

"I'm going to live as well as you do at Mayantuyacu!" the campesino spat back.

Juan's face darkened with rage, but he held his tongue, saying only, "I am your master, and I will not condemn you. But Nature itself may not forgive you."

Sandra tried to reason with him, and she finally offered to purchase the trees, paying the same price for them as the timber companies, if only they were left standing.

"It's too late," Hermano said. "I signed the contract. Go talk to them if you want." Turning his back on them, he disappeared into the darkness of his shack.

In Pucallpa, Juan and Sandra, accompanied by their lawyer, visited the regional office of the timber company. They were kept waiting, and then finally shown into the district manager's office. As Juan kneaded his hands, a Peruvian in a three-piece suit arose to greet them from behind a massive wooden desk and invited them to sit in the chairs he had arranged before him.

They sat. The man rested his elbows on the polished top of his desk, entwined his fingers, and listened as they identified themselves.

"Mayantuyacu!" he repeated. "Of course! We have been waiting to hear from you." Reaching into a drawer of his desk, he withdrew a document.

"We have an inventory of all the trees on your land, and we are ready to make you an offer."

Juan and Sandra froze. Their lawyer extended his hand. "May I see that document, please?" he asked, smiling.

"Certainly," the man smiled in return, and handed it to him.

The lawyer ripped up the document.

The man's smile disappeared.

"You had no right to this information," the lawyer stated. "This is an invasion of privacy."

"Ah, yes," the man said. "I'm not sure how we came across that document."

Juan, however, could easily imagine. Someone had been walking his land as a spy. Brusquely interrupting, he demanded: "Are you going to cut the trees around Mayantuyacu or not?"

The man looked at him, perplexed. This was not the dirt-poor campesino with dollar signs in his eyes that he had expected.

"Yes, we have signed an agreement and have begun making arrangements. . . ."

"Then it's on your head," Juan replied, and withdrew into silence.

Sandra hastily stepped in. Explaining the purpose of Mayantuyacu, she again made the offer to purchase all the trees that Hermano had sold, if only they would be left standing.

Folding his hands, the man said, "I regret very much, señora, that this will not be possible. As I said, we have already made arrangements to begin their extraction. I am very sorry."

The meeting was over. The enemy was loose inside the city walls.

Mayantuyacu, during our months there, had seemed a vast domain, where one could wander on wooded paths in all directions, undisturbed by the machines of the city. But the dream of an inaccessible Shangri-la came crashing down with the first sound of falling trees I heard from the hammock on the deck of my cabin.

We watched those carefully tended winding paths converted into rivers of mud beneath the treads of tractors. We saw the trunks of shihuahuaco, tamamuri, and lupuna trees dragged through the forest, huge as whales, to be stacked up alongside the river. In ayahuasca ceremonies, the spirits of the land came crying.

Walking out to the river one morning with Brunswick to document the devastation, I found the road once painstakingly set with white stones churned back to mud again, a giant broken cable lying discarded in the middle, the innumerable small trees and plants lining the way torn into shreds. I could not help thinking the words, "This is a sacrilege."

Descending the muddy embankment, we encountered a bright yellow tractor. I got my camera out and began taking shots of the machine, of the stacked trees, of the degradation of the landscape. At the edge of the river, I came upon the head of a *garza,* a colorful river bird I had seen flying over our launch many times. Now it lay dismembered and rotting in the mud. Nearby, its entrails lay cast off in a plastic bag. Large numbers of mosquitos now worried my skin.

Walking up to a thatched-roof shelter, I sat by the fire with Brunswick and the workers, watching an unidentified bird simmer in the pot. They made instant coffee, and we chatted politely in between the crude jokes they made at the expense of a worn-down woman who tended their camp, to which she cackled in delight. Learning that I was a professor of English, they peppered me with questions about how long it would take to acquire the magical language that offers such a leg up in the world.

These were men trapped in the cul-de-sac of *mestizaje.* Mixed-blood descendants of natives dispossessed of their ancestral terrain and culture, they eeked out an existence by participating in the destruction of the forest that had once guaranteed their freedom.

Without education, courteous and wary, prematurely old from malnutrition and a lifetime of hard labor, they were the outcome of a social agenda that reminded me of the words of a Virginian slaveholder in the antebellum United States: "We have as far as possible closed every avenue by which light may enter slaves' minds. If we could extinguish the capacity to see the light our work would be completed; they would be on a level with the beasts of the field."[10]

One of the workers commented on how his health instantly improved whenever he came out to work in the jungle, and I took the opportunity to present an alternative economic model: the trees are more valuable standing. The owners of the land need to organize and begin working their land in sustainable ways.

"Bueno, but those trees are scrap trees," he replied. "And they're dangerous because they fall down so easily. We are going to reforest with trees that are really valuable and stand up better to time."

Glancing over at the hundred-plus-year-old massive trees they had cut down, I wondered who had taught him botany.

As we returned, the photo-op I had been hoping for came crashing through the trees. A second tractor hoved into view out of the green, its front blade polished to a shine. As I stood to the side, shooting pictures as quickly as my camera would allow, I watched, puzzled, as the drivers appeared to straighten and pose for the shot. As it passed I saw clamped in its pair of mechanical jaws an entire tree. I continued shooting as the tractor fishtailed its way onward, dragging its prey in its wake.

That'll put the fear of publicity into them, I thought, stowing away my evidence.

A couple of days later news of this episode reached me through the grapevine.

The Maestro had returned to the family home in Pucallpa, and he proceeded to give an account of my visit to the encampment. Far from being alarmed by my efforts at documentation, the workers had been thrilled. The poses struck by the men on the tractor had been in honor of the Westerner who had come to photograph their labors.

The Maestro, grateful for the comic relief, gave an imitation of me, eating my liver in rage, shooting photos in every direction, while the workers preened themselves for their roles in bringing progress to the jungle. I got a glimpse of myself—the Buster Keaton of the jungle, my face grave and slightly bewildered, frantically dashing about trying to save the entire ecosystem of the Amazon basin.

It was time to take a deep breath and get some perspective for the long haul. And to start finding some allies.

10 OUR REVELS NOW ARE ENDED

A snake which gets wounded heals itself.
If now this is done by the snake, do not be
astonished for you are the snake's son. Your
father does it, and you inherit his capacity,
and therefore you are also a doctor.

PARACELSUS

I had craved the jungle in my heart of hearts ever since I began to suspect the possibility of its existence: an open system, where the daily round of eating and being eaten is supported by a hidden harmony that can be directly intuited, but never completely fathomed.

My own culture now looked solely interested in what could be captured from the known and imprisoned in boxes: whether within the four walls of a church, within the monolithic immensity of skyscrapers, or on the rectangular screen of a computer or television. Where could one drink the untrammeled freedom of the wild within such a world?

243

As the journey that had begun two years earlier in the heat-stricken Saharan antipodes of the jungle drew to a close, I felt akin to a wild animal about to be released into the middle of a financial district to fend for itself.

I also knew this was the final test—to bear the medicine back into the ordinary world and integrate it so thoroughly that no rough edges remained. The sentience of plants had to burn like a constant blue flame, a hidden pilot light, within me. Otherwise, I feared that I would dry up and suffer from phantoms of overly potent memory.

In our final week, as we quietly readied ourselves for our departure, Susana made a crown of feathers for our friend Leo, who needed some of the shaman's tools of the trade for his work. As she fashioned it she felt like an indigenous person honored with the task of preparing for an important ritual. As I sat with her watching her deft brown fingers at work, I asked her if she felt ready to leave.

"It's not really a question of leaving," she said, setting down a bright blue feather. "I belong here, my little being has its place here, so I don't feel like I'm going anywhere. I've learned that when you belong deeply to a place, you have a feeling of freedom wherever you go."

"In that case, we have to protect this land, because if we lose this wilderness we will lose our freedom. If Mayantuyacu goes, it will be like cutting out our heart," I replied.

It was in our final ceremony of ayahuasca with the Maestro that Susana's study came to its fruition. While devoting herself to analyzing the icaros and their effects on listeners, she had assiduously cultivated her relationship with chacruna in diet, entering more and more into communion with the consciousness of the plant. Seated beside her in the darkness of the maloca, I heard a melody softly arising, a music stirring within her from another realm. Then a song burst forth, coming from the pure land of the goddess Chacruna, which with a compassion surpassing human range, brushed over us and left us breathless in its wake. She had become one with the landscape of the plant, and now understood what it meant to have an icaro born from within.

She also had a vision where she saw herself pregnant and wearing a white *cushma,* the long indigenous robe of the region, although the designs woven into it were less complex than the Shipibo. She now belonged in a family way: she had joined the communion of souls within the tradition of curanderismo.

As I sat before Juan a last time in the darkness, receiving the smoke and perfume, listening to his icaros weaving the spirit worlds of the jungle, I wept in gratitude. I too felt impregnated with the virtue of Mayantuyacu. Putting my hand on his shoulder, I clasped it for a long time.

Then a cushma for Leo, woven by a local Asháninca woman, arrived the following day. Unpacking the white garment, Susana recognized in its black and red designs the same robe she had been wearing in her vision.

The morning of our departure, I awoke to the sound of Juan's flute, an enchanted melody drifting through the valley. I lay in bed listening in wonder. I had only heard him play his simple wooden flute at the end of ceremonies in the maloca. In the awakening day it was celebratory, full of good things, love of the land, praise of the spirits.

Then I realized it was the rooster crowing.

I laughed. I had come a long way from awakening in heart-racing fear to the cry of the muezzin in Fez two years before.

Later on that morning, as we cinched up our backpacks and surveyed the unnatural emptiness of our cabins, Juan appeared in full ceremonial regalia carrying a three-foot-long pipe: an exotic-looking specimen of local artesanía.

"We must all smoke together before you go," he announced. "And take a commemorative photo together."

Susana found herself assigned to put on the cushma of her vision and Leo's crown of feathers for the photo. The outfit felt completely natural to her, and in the shot she stands relaxed, the feathers of her crown glowing deep blue and brilliant red in the sun. To her left, I stand leaning lightly on a bow, looking thin as a rail in a Shipibo vest, holding arrows and squinting into the sun. Juan is laughing and wielding his pipe, and Brunswick, dressed in his best white shirt and his necklace of *encantos,* is peering at the camera with his characteristic woodland creature expression.

Doffing our costumes, we walked up to collect our bags and lingered awhile at the grave of Tigrilla. Holding hands, we descended and bid farewell to the family of workers at Mayantuyacu. Giving the Maestro an embrace, we began our hike out of the valley.

The wide Pachitea River carried us away in a plenitude of sunshine. In another photo we are seated next to each other in the launch, the features of our faces as finely cut as ancient Greek marble, our smiles porcelain, the gaze of our eyes rarified. Behind us, the smoke of burning jungle rises into the sky.

Downriver we motored, out of our awakening beneath the forest canopy, back into the vexed dream of Western civilization.

One last stop remained to make in my pilgrimage: Cuzco, the former seat of the Incan empire, high in the Andes. The art of Juan Flores owed much to the spirit of the ancient Incans, and I had yearned to walk on granite and breathe mountain air for months. Susana had already visited Cuzco numerous times and her return plane ticket was at the point of expiring, so she told me she would await my return in California a couple of weeks later.

It was to be our first separation in a year. We were threadbare and filled with uncertainty, without a home or work to return to. Our bank accounts were drained. All we had was each other and our backpacks filled with journals and recordings.

Lacing a pendant of an owl carved in green soapstone around her wrist, I embraced her in the Lima airport and told her that my life was with her. I watched her disappear behind the giant walls of frosted glass at the departure gate, and then I was alone.

It was the final days of the festival of Corpus Christi when I arrived in Cuzco, wrapped in a Shipibo cloth against the freezing air conditioning system of the bus. Finding an inexpensive hostel, I settled in and dedicated myself to writing in the cold, dark mornings, emerging to explore only when the high-altitude sun began to warm the land.

In the afternoons I watched the Cuzqueños, fortified with hits of *pisco,* heft floats of flower-laden saints onto their shoulders. Slowly maneuvering their ponderous weight out of the churches, they then launched them into the midst of the gathered populace in the Plaza de Armas. Santiago Killer of Muslims, San Sebastián pierced by arrows, the Virgin of Carmen, San Jose, the Virgin María, San Pedro, San Martín de Porres, floated triumphant, decked out in richly embroidered tunics, over the throng to the pealing of horns and the beating of drums. Wending their way to the cathedral, they "greeted" the body of Christ, embodied in the Sacred Host, kept in a gold pix standing nearly three feet tall—no doubt cast in gold once plundered from the Incan empire.

Watching the festivities reminded me of the positive side of the process of mestizaje: how it allows indigenous people to survive waves of foreign aggression to their worlds. They mix their blood and culture even while holding on to tradition, and they wait for the destructive wave to pass.

Spanish missionaries, riding the coattails of the conquistadors, had replaced the Incan mummies venerated in traditional celebrations with images of the saints. In this particular case, Tayti Inti, the Sun Father, had been deposed by Christ himself. This sleight of hand only partially succeeded. The children of the Inca refused to forget their customs: along with their traditional dances, they slyly reincorporated the features of the mummies into the images of the saints.

As I eased myself into the stream of visitors flowing through the region, I joined a tour of the Sacred Valley. Watching the other tourists clamber about in their brilliant tennis shoes, snapping photos and chattering in the disconnected way civilized people do, I appreciated even more the world of indigenous silence I had passed through in recent months. Some latent thirst for mystery had drawn them there, but without native ears and eyes, the ruins remain indecipherable.

At Sacsayhuamán—"Sexy Woman" our guide laughingly told us,

jawing the Incan words into distorted English, the great temple lying upon a high ridge a mile from Cuzco—I listened to an account of how Cuzco had been constructed in the shape of a jaguar, and how the long rows of standing stones we were facing represented the teeth in the head of the cat.

A glimpse of a now familiar cosmology, but realized on an epic scale, beckoned. My heart began to race. A cosmopolitan kingdom, a far-flung empire surpassing any of the European kingdoms of its age, whose guardian deity was the jaguar!

But then I overheard another guide describing how flying saucers had been instrumental in carrying the stones to their present locale, and my heartbeat quickly subsided. What need was there to impose exotic technological explanations upon the accomplishments of an indigenous culture that still existed? As we crossed the asphalt road to visit the shrine of Tambomachay, our dislocation in time and space only seemed to widen.

The shrine, elaborately constructed of finely carved stone, was sacred to the spirit of water, our guide informed us, and it was visited each year by the Incas in a pilgrimage to offer veneration to the element that was seen as the origin of life. At Tambomachay, two aqueducts continue to transport and maintain a constant flow of clear water during the entire year, which collects in a well the size of a large baptismal font. It was there that the Incas performed the liturgy to renew the waters throughout the land. It was there that the most exalted of human beings recognized his and his people's interconnection with the living cosmos.

We were invited to approach and rinse our mouths from this well.

As I watched groups and couples file past, I saw the dark backward abyss of time gape between our cultures. Photos snapped, hands scooped water, people smiled to commemorate the moment, but no one made an offering. The sentience of the water, which was taken for granted at Mayantuyacu, was the forgotten key element in the guide's re-creation of the pre-Hispanic world.

The sun was beginning to set behind the high cliffs when we arrived at Ollantaytambo. Climbing the terraces to the temple of the sun, where carvings of jaguars have been defaced and the rays of the sun fell upon six massive monoliths subtly set as timepieces in astronomical worship, I sat watching the colors shift in the chill, rarified sky of the Sacred Valley.

Enough tourists had cleared out to get a sense of the ruin. I smoked my pipe and sang quietly, pausing whenever little groups of tourists came through to listen to descriptions of how the great stones were transported to their present site. No one attempted to re-create the world, to summon back its deities and genius. The place was a primitive engineering marvel, nothing more. Along with the carvings of the jaguars, it appeared that all memory of the Incas had been defaced from the surface of the earth.

Then I thought of how these ruins are simply monuments to the cosmology that curanderos like Juan still uphold—how significant the meticulously laid stones appear in the light of his still living tradition. I pondered how reversed the world has become, where shamans are now the dirt-poor mestizos, when they once surrounded the royal Incas and created the brilliant rituals and sciences of medicine, astronomy, and architecture of the empire.

Remembering how often after ceremony in Mayantuyacu I had rested, contemplating the geometrical forms of the maloca, wondering whether it was an Incan temple in disguise, it was easy to speculate that the ruins I had visited that day probably had their prototypes in the otherworld, where Incan culture flourishes still.

After the tourists left a sudden torrent of goats came flowing over the rocks, followed by a goatherd caked in the dirt of the mountain, the boy's indigenous features betraying that he was more truly the owner of the mount than any other. He stopped.

"Would you like me to sing you a song in Quechua?"

"Okay," I said.

He began his song, clapping frenetically. After hearing the icaros of Juan for five months, it grated at my ears. I stopped him.

We shared a piece of chocolate together.

"*Un solcito, para mi pan. . . . ,*" he whined. Giving him a coin, I watched him disappear over the hill, following his goats.

Susana was having her own adventures. The second day of her return, caught in traffic in downtown San Francisco in a convertible with the top down, smoke suddenly began rising from beneath the hood. Pulling over, she found herself stranded on the corner of Ninth and Mission.

Her heart racing, she looked around, seeing the round canopies of trees displaced by the square profiles of buildings. The horizon had vanished. Beneath the last patch of available sky, a single straggling tree grew, past which people pushed shopping carts, talking to the air.

For the first time in months, she felt heavy isolation. Trying to soothe her fear, she cast about for a familiar referent and found her senses hitting concrete. The inter-connectivity of the life of the jungle, where each inhabitant is working in favor of the other, had receded. In its place reigned a static world, filled with traffic and people moving past in their self-absorbed inner space, their connection with one another and the world around them broken.

How can any of those moving objects offer any orientation for where you are or what you can do? she asked. *How can any of it bring you back to your center?*

Sitting for that hour it took for the engine to cool, watching the street people drift by and baking in the hot sun heavy with exhaust fumes, she felt as vulnerable as she ever had in facing Pinochet's armored storm troopers. But it was a different kind of vulnerability. She no longer feared a beating with truncheons or imprisonment and torture. She feared losing her sense of being embedded in a meaningful world.

"I felt my muscles beginning to tense back up again into the postures of self-defense I used to hold," she told me over the phone. "I felt that to live in this world, it will be necessary to make our experience of the Amazon invisible. Otherwise, it will not be possible to keep our deep relaxation in the midst of all the alertness you have to maintain here."

Listening to her story from an Internet café in Cuzco, I had an image of us carrying water in cupped hands across the frontier. How careful we would have to be not to spill the medicine we had received onto the concrete.

"I love you, Susanita," I told her. "You're the treasure of my heart. Give me a few more days and I will be back to join you."

"Bito, me too. Come home. I will be there to receive you at the airport."

And she was. Beholding her as I spilled out of the passenger gate, the high cheekbones and warm brown eyes I had come to know better than the features of my own face, I knew this was the woman I would endure through time with.

We embraced, cocooning each other.

"Robert, you're not going to believe this. Just as I was leaving Aaron's house he thrust a present for you into my hands. I'll show it to you when we get to the car."

As we threaded our way through the airport, I tried to accustom myself to the strangely transparent sound of English, and the odd textures and contours of the world I used to inhabit. I felt like a fish dropped into an aquarium. Welcome back to the bubble world. In the parking lot, Susana swung open the door of the car and reached in. Pulling out a folded T-shirt, she said, "This is your present."

Unfurling it like a flag, she revealed the image of a puma.

People tended to have two versions of me upon my return. The first came from my father.

My old truck had been sitting abandoned beneath a tree, through four seasons of Sierra mountain weather, filling with spiders and dust. I had to get it started; my father offered me a lift to it. When we met at the El Cerrito BART station, he looked surprised as I climbed into the car.

"You look good. I almost didn't recognize you when I pulled up. I thought you'd have long hair and a beard."

"And be wearing a jaguar skin, huh?"

"Well, I didn't know what to expect. You've been gone a long time."

I could feel my father's uncertainty over what had become of his son.

"I got my hair cut in Cuzco for half a buck. You know, living in the jungle can actually be pretty civilized. Just because we didn't have electricity doesn't mean we were living in trees."

He scrutinized me. "You look better than I've ever seen you, actually."

This was an interesting comment, considering the fact I looked like I had just survived forty days and forty nights in the desert.

"Whatever you did there, it suits you pretty well. But you're going to have to start eating again."

As we drove he caught me up on the news of the family. From my side, there was only so much I could relate to him about our lives in the jungle, but as the car left Highway 80 and started winding along the country roads into the mountains, I announced that I had a story to tell him.

Taking a deep breath, I narrated the events of the ceremony at Mayantuyacu wherein I had returned to the womb and re-experienced the intrusion that had disrupted my development as a fetus. My father sat listening, rapt.

I then laid out how that intrusion had set up the conditions for the angry rebellion that had driven me onto the streets as a child. I knew, of course, that the bigger picture included the family dynamics I was born into, but I didn't mention those, or the underlying connection between my psychomachia and the short life of my brother.

As I spoke, there was a resonance in the car, as if I was laying bare some ancient, obscure design woven into our family history. Concluding my tale, I awaited his response. It looked as if some weight had just been lifted from his shoulders. "I don't believe a word of it," he finally said with a sigh. "But I've never heard anything that explains what happened in our family better."

The other picture I got was from various friends, many of whom also couldn't recognize me. I looked like a walking skeleton, I heard through the grapevine, and seemed spacey and disconnected. When I tried to relate my journey, I felt like the ancient mariner clutching the arm of the wedding guest. Old friends interrupted my narrative with crude jokes or changed the subject.

I had been gone too long and had traveled too far. People seemed tuned in to a radio channel that played day and night in their heads, and I couldn't hear it.

But we found the work with the plants had forged little inroads to the culture, which proved crucial, and enduring. We located our house on a hilltop in Oakland when the owner recognized our connection with her garden, and one of my best teaching positions opened for me after I had already given my pitch over the phone and been turned down. My interviewer still seemed open, however, so I told him about the work that we had been doing in the Amazon. In the middle of my description, he interrupted me and asked, "So, were you doing ayahuasca down there?"

I took a risk. "Yes, it's very much part of that culture."

"My friends have always told me I should try that." There was a moment of silence, and then he said, "Well, why don't you come in? We might have something for you after all."

As Susana settled into an analysis of two hundred pages worth of interviews, I commenced the life of a highway flier on the gritty freeways encircling the San Francisco Bay. I felt like a marble set rolling in a metal bowl. As the weeks passed into months, I found the amplification of my senses that the jungle had permitted wasn't subsiding. The world turned gray as I cut myself down to a standard part that could fit back into the economic machine. I became depressed. Even worse, I lost my ability to write.

Joseph Campbell, that great explicator of the hero's journey, taught that one variant in the hero's return was that the medicine turns into a handful of dust as soon as the hero steps out of the forest. There were days returning from my long hours of teaching when I felt so empty I wondered if I had failed in my quest.

Yes, I had heard the voice of Yahweh naming the creatures of the world and identified the error that lay behind the metaphysics of the West: the voice that awoke our ancestors from slumber was not an abstract power lying above and beyond the Creation. It was the Garden itself. We *are* Nature.

But that and a buck fifty can get me a cup coffee, I thought. *The daylight world isn't interested in the goings-on of the otherworld.*

I began perversely wishing I could reinsert myself into the snug world of the American dream again. It began to sink in that I had, as so many others before, sought the answers for my life in the realm of the dead, and I was now facing the consequences. The etymology of the word *ayahuasca*—the vine of the dead, which I had taken only half-seriously— was as faithful to its reality as any word woven out of human experience could be.

Pondering this issue of transplantation, a story came back to me of the humble curandero in the little town of Chazuta who, it was discovered, had been successfully healing leprosy with a little plant called Shishinto. A German pharmaceutical company, hearing about the possible resolution of this ancient blight upon humanity, rushed in and secured the method of preparation from him. But then after rigorously duplicating the curandero's recipe, they found the medicine ineffective. Returning to Chazuta, they asked the curandero, "What went wrong? How could it be that when we followed exactly the same stages of preparation as you, the medicine doesn't work?"

"Oh," the curandero laughed. "You didn't sing to the plant! Without the icaro, the medicine doesn't work."

I began to wonder if the medicine had abandoned me. Perhaps I had never truly grasped it in the first place.

Then one night as I lay dreaming in bed next to Susana, my spirit wandered through a warehouse store blazing with fluorescent light, severe with rows of goods honed down to their plastic and garish minimum. Seeking a way out of this new morph of the Wal-Mart concept, I encountered a black metal gate extending in both directions, upon which was mounted a sign that commanded:

FIX IN YOUR MIND THAT **YOURSTORE** OFFERS YOU THE
BEST VALUE AND LOWEST PRICE FOR YOUR DOLLAR!

Wow, I thought. *Advertising has sure been losing its subtlety in my absence.*

Finally seeing a guard, I asked him how to exit and he pointed to a little door in the metal wall. Passing through, I was surprised to find Brunswick outside on the sidewalk with an older Indian man. Standing with a cup before him, Brunswick was singing icaros for spare change.

"What's he doing here?" I wondered out loud.

A voice answered dismissively, "Oh, he's always standing there singing."

The older Indian stood silently, wrapped in a poncho and wearing a conical felt hat. His deep brown eyes just watched. Suddenly recognizing him, I turned to him and bowing, said, "I owe you for the medicine. Please allow me to offer you something for the gift."

"No," the old man said, smiling and shaking his head. "You owe me nothing. The medicine is yours."

I awoke still feeling the numinous presence of that old indio, and I knew then that I had made it home with the medicine after all.

Susana and I were married on December 8, the day of the Buddha's enlightenment and the Immaculate Conception of the Virgin Mary, symbolically uniting our two faiths in a single union.

The ceremony was a civil one, conducted in the City Hall of San Francisco. Both of my parents were present, and my mother comforted me as I walked, close to tears, behind my bride to register our names with the county clerk. Susana's parents awaited news and photos in Chile.

In a small ecumenical chapel we exchanged our vows, to cherish and hold each other as long as we lived. An orchestra was playing that day within the lavish art deco interior of the main hall, and afterward we danced across the marble floors as our friends snapped photos and applauded from the balcony above. As we descended the outer steps of City Hall, a policeman, seeing us coming, walked briskly into the center of the crosswalk and halted the oncoming traffic in our honor.

It suddenly felt good to be home in the city I loved.

Across the street in the plaza, beneath the trailing legs of a surrealistic animal sculpture scavenged from Burning Man, our friends had prepared a more intimate ritual for us. There they summoned our ancestors and, putting brooms in our hands, had us sweep away any obscurations lying in our family lineages. A member of the Native American Church appeared to call blessings from the four directions upon us.

"Are we really married?" Susana asked in the car driving to the restaurant. "I thought I'd feel different when I got married, but I don't. Do you think it's real?" She turned to me with a worried look.

"As far as I'm concerned it is."

"I never wanted to get married anyway. All those years and all those opportunities that I turned down. I wanted to be free, not trapped in a role."

Now I was getting worried. "You're still free. We haven't locked ourselves into a role, instead we've made commitments to one another within which our relationship can evolve. It's a practice, not a set of expectations.

"Besides," I added, "maybe it doesn't feel like anything different because we already were married, joined in the dragon's blood, as it were. We've simply made it public."

"Okay," she brightened. "I can live with that."

And we have.

Dr. Susana Bustos's study of icaros has borne fruit both academically and personally. Her dissertation is being received as an eloquent and theoretically incisive work on a little-understood subject. Her songs continue to blossom forth from the marirí of chacruna.

The jaguar still rumbles within me, and at times I can sense her gaze flickering luminously behind mine, as if she still stalks my inner psyche, but her spirit appears little interested in northern cities or dry mountain regions of pine, madrone, and oak. She basically retired from view on our return, although she surges back to life whenever we have taken groups of pilgrims down to Mayantuyacu to experience work with the plants with the Maestro Juan Flores.

Then we have our reunion in the world of spirit, and our ancient bond is always there.

> *Be not afeard. The isle is full of noises,*
> *Sounds, and sweet airs, that give delight and hurt not.*
> *Sometimes a thousand, twangling instruments*
> *Will hum about mine ears, and sometimes voices*
> *That, if I then had waked after long sleep,*
> *Will make me sleep again; and then, in dreaming,*
> *The clouds methought would open and show riches*
> *Ready to drop upon me, that when I waked*
> *I cried to dream again.*
>
> SHAKESPEARE, *THE TEMPEST*

ACKNOWLEDGMENTS

With gratitude I wish to recognize the entire web of relations that aided in the bringing forth of this book. I especially wish to thank Robert Aitken Roshi and Nelson Foster for their years of guidance in the Way, as well as William Merwin, who first opened my eyes to the sentience of nature and how "the whole of life is necessary for the whole of life."

Other generous spirits with whom I have had illuminating talks or at whose hands I have received succor are Louis Bluecloud, Sheelo Bohm, Débora Bolsanello, Julia Caban, Judyth Collin, Robert and Meg Ellis, Lia Gatey, Sean Kerrigan, Lorna Li, Maryann Lipaj, Jeremy Narby, Dale and Laura Pendell, Jen Sheffield, Gary Snyder, Kent Tindall, Pat Walsh, and Brad Yantzer.

To the scientific pioneers Philippe Bandeira de Melo of the Arca da Criacão and Jacques Mabit and Rosa Giove of the Centro Takiwasi, as well as the communities of Daime in Brazil, in gratitude for their welcome and for their endeavors to transmit the ancient ways of the rain forest to the modern world.

Finally, and above all, I wish to thank the master curandero Juan Flores Salazar and his partner, Sandra Encalada Guerra, for their welcome to Mayantuyacu. We arrived virtually penniless, and they put more water in the soup so we could stay.

THE VERSE OF THE PLANT WE FOLLOW

Susana Bustos, Ph.D.

> *The genie of the plant is tiny. It teaches you the verses . . .*
> *It makes you hear when you sleep, continues with the verse*
>   *as you copy it . . .*
> *The verse remains in your body and continues completing*
>   *with time.*
> *He who has completed his verse can sing. There they*
>   *direct . . .*
> *The verse of the plant we follow, of the plant, of its*
>   *medicine.*
>
>   DON GUILLERMO, MAESTRO CURANDERO

To try to answer the question of how icaros work and heal is as complex as addressing the phenomenon of music itself: whatever standpoint one takes always seems a fragment of the proverbial elephant. Peruvian Amazonian *vegetalistas,* embedded in a particular cosmological understanding and experience of reality, hold these types of shamanic songs in ways that stretch our usual Western minds into archaic territories. Let's first listen to their voices in this polyphonic approach to the icaros.

HEALERS' VOICES

Through the icaros the "others" act,
one attracts the force of the plant.

DON ORLANDO

Peruvian mestizo curanderos or vegetalistas utilize these songs in most of their practices, such as when fishing and hunting particular species, protecting themselves or others, gaining the love of a woman through magical arts, infusing objects or persons with particular powers for healing or sorcery, and activating the powers of medicinal compounds by invoking and praising their powers (Luna 1986, 1992; Bustos 2005). During ayahuasca rituals, the ayahuasquero employs icaros to set a beneficial and secure spiritual space for himself and for his or her clients' journey, and to effectively act upon the clients' health issues and experiences while they are under the influence of the brew.

When one asks a curandero how he works with the icaros, he may simply answer: "It's the genie of the plant who does the job, not me." Many of them may add that a humble, loving, and praising attitude while singing is what the spirits require from them in order not to interfere with the spirits' work and to be receptive to their instructions. Some curanderos also believe that singing stimulates and directs the work of the invoked powers toward a specific goal (Bustos 2005, 2006).

In fact, the curandero has gained the favor of the powers he deals with through a long and hard training phase that consists of dieting brews made out of plants, minerals, or other substances. The genie of the plant then comes to him in dreams or dreamlike states to cure—and to teach him its secrets about how to empower himself, gain skills, and cure. The culmination of the blessing is the reception of the icaro, the very essence of that power.

Along with the phlegm or mariri of the plants that accumulate in the chest of the curandero through the dieting process, which constitutes one of his main defenses against bad spirits, the icaros hold a double nature: they have material and immaterial qualities (Luna and Amaringo 1991). When the diet and the training are correctly pursued, the songs end up inserted into the physical and energetic structure of the healer's mind/body, from which the healer acquires the right resonance to sing them and activate their powers (Jacques Mabit in Bustos 2006). Rosa Giove tells the story of don Solón, an old and prestigious curandero, now in his nineties, who was in sharp and enduring back pain when he asked her for Western medical help. When she didn't find anything anomalous in his back, he smiled and said: "Oh, it may then be just an icaro that came out of place."

The icaros are not always received through diets: they can be also transmitted from teacher to apprentice by following a similar installment procedure into the prepared mind/body of the apprentice. In this case, the teacher sings the icaro onto the top of the apprentice's head and into his body, a process that can last several days or even weeks, and is helped by blowing tobacco smoke and perfumes over him, as well as by beating the shacapa on him (Jacques Mabit in Bustos 2006). Sometimes healers receive icaros during ayahuasca ceremonies or in their dreams at night. Or they may learn icaros from one another, or compose them when they have gained enough experience as healers. However, the most powerful icaros are considered the ones received directly from the plants. These usually come in tongues, or in Quichua, a Quechua dialect from the area (Luna 1986).

WESTERN VOICES

"I would say that the reason music [in ayahuasca experiences] has such a special psychological impact is precisely because it is abstract . . . and at the same time very concrete . . . this coupling of the abstract and the concrete is a characteristic of human cognition in general" (Shanon 2002, 311).

To the Western ear the icaros may sound repetitive and monotonous, even given the heightened sensitivity that is opened by the effects of the ayahuasca. Their tempo is usually constant, above the normal range of the human heartbeat, in a binary rhythm. Their melody is most often built on a pentatonic scale, with short motifs of small intervals that repeat over and over again. The lyrics of the icaros, on the other hand, are usually short phrases within long repetitive syllables—*trananais, denderendes, rarararais*—that have no apparent meaning (Bustos 2008; Brabec 2002). However, a closer listening and musical analysis reveal dozens of minimal melodic and rhythmic variations, as well as subtle expressive and text differences in the lyrics, which are almost never the same across ceremonies. It seems as if an icaro is re-created anew every time a shaman sings it, even if it sounds as if it's the same song to the listener.

Niemeyer, a Brazilian anthropologist who has studied the lyrics of ayahuasca songs of indigenous tribes, presents an interesting argument about their multiple variations, applicable to the melodic variations of the icaros. While it is well known that the psyche of a shaman at work is scissionned into different dimensions that are simultaneously available to experience in the here and now, Niemeyer states that the song reflects their stereoscopic synthesis. The basic structure of the lyrics of a song sets a prescribed spiritual path for the shaman to undertake, which is safe for him and culturally legitimized, yet his particular journey varies every time. Insofar as this is concerned, he incorporates in the lyrics bits of his own journey into these archetypal realms, bits of his experience of the spiritual and concrete realities of the ceremony he is holding, and bits of the situation and issues he sees in the patient. Therefore, these songs can never be sung in exactly the same way each time; they provide a structure that may only make complete sense to the shaman himself as he follows and re-creates it in the uniqueness of each particular setting.

If we now put ourselves in the position of a client, with or without the influence of the ayahuasca brew, we notice that the characteristics of these songs can have an entrancing effect on our psyches. Their repetitious quality may be particularly soothing under ayahuasca in that they anchor the person's experience into familiar patterns, which additionally offer alternative pathways for the activated archetypal psyche to follow.

In this way, the icaros contribute in the structuring of the experience (see also Katz and de Rios 1971). Nonetheless, the person is simultaneously functioning at different depths of awareness as deep unconscious material presses to make its way to the conscious psyche. It is then possible to understand how the subliminal variations are capable of highly enriching the alternatives for that material to configure itself into form. These forms manifest as new perspectives on old issues never seen before, deep insights, visions of unknown territories, encounters with archetypal beings or dead people, and mystical experiences, as well as many other unusual experiences.

But what is the experience of a person who undergoes an intense healing with an icaro during these rituals?

CLIENTS' VOICES

When I hear someone with such a calm voice, singing
for you, in a situation like this: an icaro, in a session, the
ayahuasca in myself . . . I think I receive, it's like I received
the energy he is passing, of calm, listening only to what he is
singing, nothing else.

A CLIENT WHO HAS UNDERGONE AN EXPERIENCE
OF INTENSE HEALING WITH AN ICARO

For vegetalistas, during an ayahuasca ceremony, the brew, the healing icaros, and the spirits do effective work whether or not the client can consciously perceive their actions or effects at the time. As it appears in my study on intense healing experiences attributed to icaros during an ayahuasca ceremony, for a client to distinctly feel that an icaro is providing healing during a ceremony is experienced as a remarkable event, and something that tends to occur only once in a while (Bustos 2008). When present, this awareness appears dependent upon several conditions of bodily preparation, mind set, and ritual setting. Maestro Juan explains that the icaros are repeated several times during ceremonies, but there is a moment when the spirits, the healer, and the patient are aligned in such a way that the person is able to feel the healing coming *through* the icaro. A client who experienced intense healing with an icaro said: "I guess another person [in the ceremony] may not have even listened to this icaro, or didn't consider it, or was there and said: ah, a new icaro! But . . . it was like if the Maestro had taken my shoulder and would have whispered to me, like: take it, this is for you, work, connect, open up. . . . And it was demolishing, because as it was, it entered where it had to."

Here let me address only a few of the constituents of this complex phenomenon: the client enters a state where the sense of self feels locked in deep absorption in the singing and the concomitant display of visions, organic sensations, emotions, and thoughts, all unfolding together in perfect syntony. The perfection of this syntonic unfoldment is described by one participant: "It was like the icaro was singing me." This moment is one of profound intimacy with oneself and with the singing, in that the client feels he is finally touching and is being touched in his core healing issue with a depth, care, and precision he has never experienced before. "It was touching me in a place that I can't give a location for, but . . . felt, or I knew, was essential, and so . . . I was in the session for that. That's what I came all the way to the Amazon for . . . to be healed." A sense of genuineness emerges as the mind and the body experience a release of old habits and patterns, and they restructure into wider and more flexible ways of being in the world. "The feeling with the icaro was that it was resolving the issue: the anger, the jealousy, the other things I brought into the session were melting as ossified things that were in my mind. Like I was being washed [of them] and the attachment to them." I call this stage of the process *communion:* communion with the singing (which embodies the otherness), communion with oneself, and communion with one's larger identity and possibilities, all of which take place during an eternal moment of glimpsing into the Mystery.

The territories that icaros cross in order to bring healing are various and subtle, palpable and ethereal; they can be partly understood by Western approaches and partly not. The fact is that the healing reaches deeply into the souls of the ones who experience it and a transformation occurs. It may be that the spirits, the effects of the plants, the influence of the curandero on the client, and the physical and psychological properties of the songs all work together in a collaborative dance orchestrated by the verse of the plant they follow.

References

Brabec, B. 2002. Ikaro: Medizinische Gesaenge der Ayawaska-Zeremonie im Peruanischen Regenwald. Unpublished master's thesis, Universitaet Wien, Austria.

Bustos, S. 2005. Icaros: El poder sanador de los curanderos amazónicos. *Revista Uno Mismo* 190:50–57.

Bustos, S. 2006. The house that sings: The therapeutic use of icaros at Takiwasi. *Shaman's Drum* 73:32–38.

Bustos, S. 2008. The healing power of the icaros: A phenomenological study of ayahuasca experiences. Unpublished doctoral dissertation, California Institute of Integral Studies, San Francisco.

Katz, F., and de Rios, M. 1971. Hallucinogenic music: An analysis of the role of whistling in Peruvian ayahuasca sessions. *Journal of American Folklore* 84(333): 320–27.

Luna, L. E. 1986. Vegetalismo: Shamanism among the mestizo population of the Peruvian Amazon. *Stockholm studies in comparative religion,* vol. 27. Stockholm: Almqvist & Wiksell International.

Luna, L. E. 1992. Magical melodies among the mestizo shamans of the Peruvian Amazon. In E. J. Langdon, *Portals of power: Shamanism in South America,* 231–53. Albuquerque: University of New Mexico Press.

Luna, L. E., & Amaringo, P. 1991. *Ayahuasca visions: The religious iconography of a Peruvian shaman.* Berkeley: North Atlantic Books.

Niemeyer, P. C. de. 2006. De duplos e estereoscópios: Paralelismo e personificacao nos cantos xamanísticos ameríndios. *Mana: Estudos de Antropologia Social* 12(1): 105–34.

Shanon, B. 2002. *The antipodes of the mind: Charting the phenomenology of the ayahuasca experience.* New York: Oxford University Press.

NOTES

Chapter 2. The Jaguar that Roams the Mind

1. Bustos, "The Healing Power of the Icaros, a Phenomenological Study of Ayahuasca Experiences."
2. Ibid.
3. Ibid.
4. Ibid.
5. White, "Supreme Court Ruling," 4–7.

Chapter 3. Fear No Spirits

1. Narby, *The Cosmic Serpent*, 38–39.
2. Plotkin, *Medicine Quest*, 29.
3. Lagrou, "Two Ayahuasca Myths," 31–35.
4. Heaney, *Over Nine Waves*, 11.

Chapter 4. Close to the Hurt Lies Growing the Balm

1. Mabit, "Blending Traditions," 25–32.
2. www.ibogaine.org/lotsof.html.
3. Plotkin, *Medicine Quest*, 21.
4. Bustos, 14.
5. Mabit, "Blending Traditions," 25–32.
6. Giove, *La Liana de los Muertos al Rescate de la Vida*, 175–77.
7. Segal, *Introduction to the Work of Melanie Klein*.
8. Narby and Huxley, *Shamans through Time*, 302.
9. Ibid., 303.

Chapter 5. The Spirit of Mist

1. Martin, "Woven Songs of the Amazon."
2. Dobkin de Rios, "Curing with Ayahuasca in an Urban Slum," 76.
3. Dobkin de Rios, "Mea Culpa." 20.
4. Von Strassburg, *Tristan,* 161.

Chapter 6. The Sacred City

1. Freedman, "The Jaguar Who Would Not Say Her Prayers," 113.
2. Ibid.
3. Siegel, *Intoxication,* 83–84.
4. Narby, *The Cosmic Serpent,* 120.
5. Hillman, *The Dream and the Underworld,* 104–5.
6. Ibid., 98–99.

Chapter 7. The Will to Heal Is the Will to Be Whole

1. Thévet, "Ministers of the Devil Who Learn About the Secrets of Nature," *Shamans Through Time,* 13.
2. Petrovich, "The Shaman: A Villian of a Magician Who Calls Demons," *Shamans Through Time,* 18.
3. Lafitau, "The Savages Esteem Their Jugglers," *Shamans Through Time,* 23.
4. Diderot and Colleagues, "Shamans Are Imposters Who Claim They Consult the Devil—And Who Are Sometimes Close to the Mark," *Shamans Through Time,* 32.
5. Gmelin, Johann Georg, "Shamans Deserve Perpetual Labor for Their Hocus-Pocus," *Shamans Through Time,* 27.
6. See Gary Snyder's essay "The Etiquette of Freedom," in his *The Practice of the Wild* for an insightful discussion into the career of Alvar Núñez Cabeza de Vaca, 15.
7. Ibid., 24.
8. Ibid.
9. Ibid.
10. Ibid.
11. Ibid.
12. Frankl, *Man's Search for Meaning,* 77–78.

13. Maloof, "Old Growth Air," *Terrain.org. A Journal of the Built and Natural Environments.*

14. Ibid.

15. Ibid.

16. Ibid.

Chapter 8. A Sweet Odor Shall Enter Their Bones

1. Mabit, Parisian lecture, 2003.

2. Luna, "The Concept of Plants as Teachers Among Four Mestizo Shamans of Iquitos, Northeastern Peru," 135–56.

3. Ibid.

4. Freedman, "The Jaguar Who Would Not Say Her Prayers," 117–18.

5. Grossinger, *Planet Medicine.*

6. Ibid.

7. Ibid.

8. Ibid, 157.

9. Ibid.

10. Narby, *Intelligence in Nature,* 50.

11. Ibid.

12. Dupré, *Passage to Modernity,* 70–74.

13. Ibid.

14. Tarnas, *Cosmos and Psyche,* 35.

Chapter 9. The Holy Tree

1. Diamond, *Guns, Germs, and Steel,* 77.

2. Ibid., 90.

3. www.Amazonwatch.org.

4. Ibid.

5. Langewiesche, "Jungle Law," 226.

6. Langewiesche, "Jungle Law."

7. Ibid.

8. www.Amazonwatch.org. Collyns, "Indigenous Amazonian People Score Rare Victory Against Oil Company."

9. Shoumatoff, "The Gasping Forest," 272–87.

10. Lovell, *Black Song: The Forge and the Flame,* 164.

BIBLIOGRAPHY

Anonymous. The Book of Enoch. Translated by Richard Laurence, LL.D. Oxford: Oxford.

Bustos, Susana. "The Healing Power of Icaros, a Phenomenological Study of Ayahuasca Experiences." Ph.D. diss., California Institute for Integral Studies, 2007.

Collyns, Dan. "Indigenous Amazonian People Score Rare Victory Against Oil Company." *The Guardian,* November 26, 2006.

Davis, Wade. *One River.* New York: Simon and Schuster, 1996.

Diamond, Jared. *Guns, Germs, and Steel.* New York: Norton, 1999.

Diderot and Colleagues. "Shamans Are Imposters Who Claim They Consult the Devil—And Who Are Sometimes Close to the Mark." In *Shamans Through Time: 500 Years on the Path to Knowledge,* edited by Jeremy Narby and Francis Huxley. New York: Jeremy P. Tarcher/Putnam, 2001.

Dobkin de Rios, Marlene. "Curing with Ayahuasca in an Urban Slum" from *Hallucinogens and Shamanism*, edited by Michael Harner. New York: Oxford University Press, 1973.

———. "Mea Culpa: Drug Tourism, and the Anthropologist's Responsibility." *Anthropology News* 47, no. 7 (October 2006): 20.

Dupré, Louis. *Passage to Modernity.* New Haven: Yale University Press, 1993.

Frankl, Viktor. *Man's Search for Meaning.* New York: Simon and Schuster, 1984.

Freedman, Françoise Barbira. "The Jaguar Who Would Not Say Her Prayers." In *The Ayahuasca Reader,* edited by Luis Eduardo Luna and Steven White. Santa Fe: Synergetic Press, 2000.

Giove, Rosa. *La Liana de los Muertos al Rescate de la Vida.* Tarapoto, Peru: Takiwasi, 2002.

Gmelin, Johnn Georg. "Shamans Deserve Perpetual Labor for Their Hocus-Pocus." In *Shamans Through Time: 500 Years on the Path to Knowledge,* edited by Jeremy Narby and Francis Huxley. New York: Jeremy P. Tarcher/Putnam, 2001.

Grossinger, Richard. *Planet Medicine*. New York: Anchor Press, 1980.

Heaney, Marie. *Over Nine Waves*. London: Faber and Faber, 1995.

Hillman, James. *The Dream and the Underworld*. New York: Harper and Row, 1979.

Lafitau, Joseph François. "The Savages Esteem Their Jugglers." In *Shamans Through Time: 500 Years on the Path to Knowledge*, edited by Jeremy Narby and Francis Huxley. New York: Jeremy P. Tarcher/Putnam, 2001.

Lagrou, Elsje Maria. "Two Ayahuasca Myths from the Cashinahua of Northwestern Brazil." In *The Ayahuasca Reader*, edited by Luis Eduardo Luna and Steven White. New Mexico: Synergetic Press, 2000.

Langewiesche, William. "Jungle Law." *Vanity Fair*, May 2007.

Lovell, John. *Black Song: The Forge and the Flame*. New York: Macmillan, 1972.

Luna, Luis Eduardo. "The Concept of Plants as Teachers Among Four Mestizo Shamans of Iquitos, Northeastern Peru." *The Journal of Ethnopharmacology* 11 (1984): 135–56.

Mabit, Jacques. "Blending Traditions: Using Indigenous Medicinal Knowledge to Treat Drug Addiction." *MAPS, Bulletin of the Multidisciplinary Association for Psychedelic Studies* 12, no. 2 (2002): 25–32.

———. Lecture given at the Centre Savoir Psy., Paris. September, 2003.

Maloof, Joan. "Old Growth Air." In *Terrain.org. A Journal of the Built and Natural Environments*, www.terrain.org/articles/14/maloof.htm.

Martin, Barrett H. "Woven Songs of the Amazon." Paper presented at the 50th Anniversary Conference of the Society for Ethnomusicology. November 2005.

Menon, Ramesh. *The Ramayana*. New York: North Point Press, 2003.

Merton, Thomas. "The Sacred City." In *Ishi Means Man*. Greensboro: Unicorn Press, 1976.

Narby, Jeremy. *The Cosmic Serpent*. New York: Jeremy P. Tarcher/Putnam, 1999.

———. *Intelligence in Nature*. New York: Tharcher/Penguin, 2005.

Narby, Jeremy, and Francis Huxley, eds. *Shamans through Time: 500 Years on the Path to Knowledge*. New York: Jeremy P. Tarcher/Putnam, 2001.

Neihardt, John. *Black Elk Speaks*. Lincoln: University of Nebraska Press, 1995.

Pendell, Dale. *Pharmakodynamis*. San Francisco: Mercury House, 2002.

Petrovich, Avvakum. "The Shaman: A Villian of a Magician Who Calls Demons." In *Shamans Through Time: 500 Years on the Path to Knowledge*, edited by Jeremy Narby and Francis Huxley. New York: Jeremy P. Tarcher/Putnam, 2001.

Plotkin, Mark. *Medicine Quest*. New York: Viking, 2000.

Segal, Hanna. *Introduction to the Work of Melanie Klein*. New York: Basic Books, 1964.

Shoumatoff, Alex. "The Gasping Forest." *Vanity Fair,* May 2007.

Siegel, Ronald. *Intoxication.* New York: Simon and Schuster, 1989.

Snyder, Gary. *The Practice of the Wild.* Washington, D.C.: Shoemaker & Hoard, 2004.

Strassman, Rick. *DMT: The Spirit Molecule.* Rochester, Vt.: Park Street Press, 2001.

Tarnas, Richard. *Cosmos and Psyche.* New York: Viking, 2006.

Thévet, André. "Ministers of the Devil Who Learn About the Secrets of Nature." In *Shamans Through Time: 500 Years on the Path to Knowledge,* edited by Jeremy Narby and Francis Huxley. New York: Jeremy P. Tarcher/Putnam, 2001.

Thoreau, Henry David. *The Portable Thoreau.* New York: Penguin Books, 1975.

Von Strassburg, Gottfried. *Tristan.* Baltimore: Penguin Books, 1965.

White, Timothy. "Supreme Court Ruling Reaffirms RFRA and the Religious Right to Use Sacraments." *Shaman's Drum* 72 (2006).

www.Amazonwatch.org.

INDEX

Page numbers followed by an "n" indicate footnotes.